THE GABRIEL METHOD

Super Delicious, Super Nutritious

RECIPE BOOK

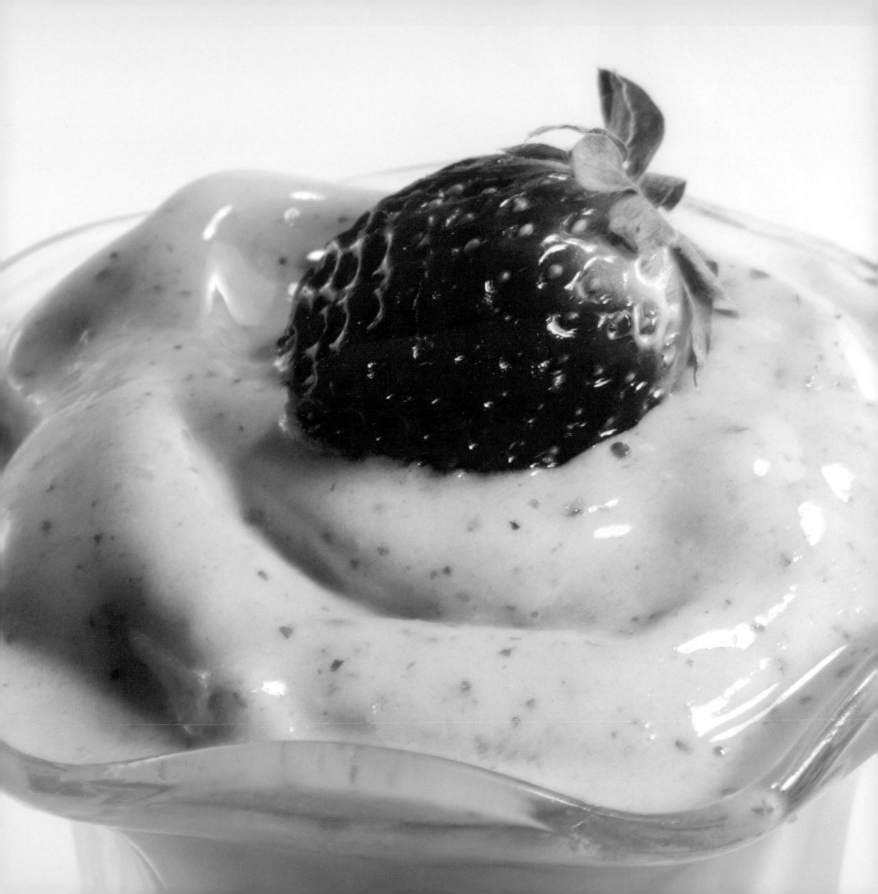

THE GABRIEL METHOD

Super Delicious, Super Nutritious

RECIPE BOOK

The Gabriel Method
Super Delicious, Super Nutritious
Recipe Book

Published in Australia by:
The Gabriel Method Pty.
Shop 8
Palm Court
Strickland Street
Denmark WA, 6333
www.TheGabrielMethod.com

Jon Gabriel
www.TheGabrielMethod.com
Email: Jon@gabrielmethod.com

Library of Congress Cataloging-in-publication data
Gabriel, Jon The Gabriel Method / Jon Gabriel ISBN - 978-0-646-56263-6

(Hardcover) 1. Health 2. Physical Fitness 3.Parenting and Children

Cover Design by Kelly Jones, i4design

Executive Editor - Xavier Waterkeyn
Assitant Editor - Lydia Kenyon

Book Design - Kelly Jones, i4design and Xavier Waterkeyn

Cover photo and some lifestyle photos - Nic Duncan
Food phototography - Oona Mansour
Food stylists - Oona Mansour and Teegan O'Hehir
Seminar photos - Jack Strom

Printed by Leo Paper Group

Disclaimer
This book is written as a source of information only. Neither the publisher nor the author are engaged in rendering medical advice to the individual reader. The information contained in this book should by no means be considered a substitute for advice of a qualified medical professional, who should always be consulted before beginning any new diet, exercise or health program. Every effort has been made to insure the accuracy of the information in this book. The author and the publisher expressly disclaim responsibility for any adverse effects arising from the use or application of the information contained herein.

To the hundreds of thousands of students we have all over the world...
you continue to inspire me daily.

Contents

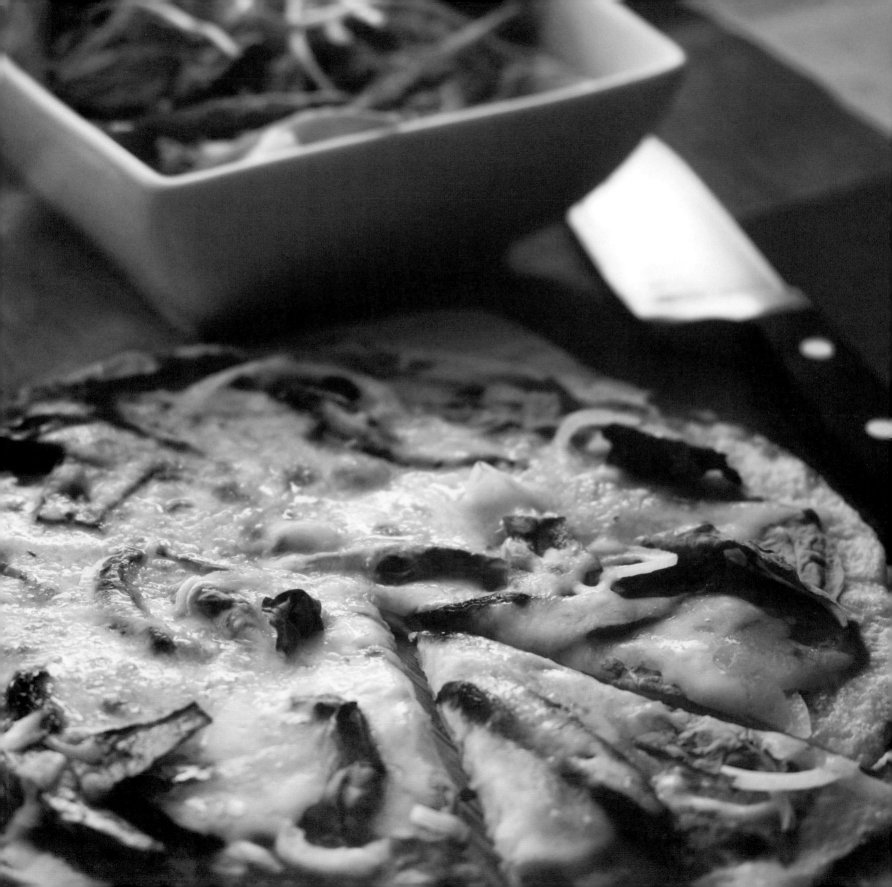

Introduction

Ever since we launched *The Gabriel Method* in 2007 there's been an overwhelmingly positive response to this radical and revolutionary approach to weightloss. After all, what other weightloss approach actually starts by asking you to *add* food!

The effectiveness of the Method has now been established through thousands of cases and documented in thousands of testimonials. Yet, from the very beginning, people have been asking us a fundamental question:

'Just how do we apply *The Gabriel Method* principles in a simple and easy to understand way specifically to the foods that we eat?'

Or to phrase it more simply:

'We want a cook book!'

Well now after eight years of passionate research into finding ways to make super healthy foods taste great, and after two further years of testing hundreds of different recipes and hundreds of hours of collating, writing and designing, here it is.

If you are new to *The Gabriel Method* let's be clear from the beginning, The Gabriel Method is not a diet. Diets work on the faulty premise that calorie restriction alone is the long-term solution to obesity. Unfortunately our bodies, as well as our hearts and minds, just don't work that way. If they did, then there'd only be one calorie-restrictive diet that would work for everyone.

Dieting Makes You Fat

Dieting doesn't address the *real* causes of obesity. In fact, restrictive dieting can actually get your body to want to be fatter because, as far as your body is concerned, 'dieting' and 'starvation' are the same thing, and when your body is starving it activates a primal starvation response that causes your body to want to hold onto weight. I call this primary response to starvation the FAT Programs. Those of you who have read *The Gabriel Method* know all about the FAT programs and how they can force you to gain weight. But for those who haven't, here's a brief summary.

When your FAT programs are activated certain subtle chemical changes take place in your body that make you hungrier, make you crave more fattening foods, slow your metabolism and put your body into a kind of perpetual fat storage mode.

Calorie restriction, or starvation, might cause you to lose weight in the short term, but as your hunger increases and your metabolism decreases, the rate at which you lose weight begins to slow. Your body is conflicted and 'fights' you and you struggle every step of the way because it thinks it is in a famine. Eventually, you stop losing weight altogether, as your body does everything it can to store every available calorie.

Once the FAT programs are activated you are in the unfortunate position of having to continue to diet, not to lose weight, but to simply maintain your current weight, all the while fighting hunger cravings day and night. Then, as you're discouraged and dejected, there will invariably come a time when you're just too tired to fight anymore. You give in to an overwhelming need to eat and you have a big binge. Weight, that's taken you weeks or even months to take off, comes back in a matter of days and the whole diet roller-coaster ride starts all over again.

Dieting isn't the only thing that can activate your FAT programs. Any form of 'starvation' such as sleep deprivation and dehydration; any form of stress such as chemical toxicity in the form of pesticides, medication, artificial sweeteners and flavour enhancers, or any emotional or mental stress can potentially activate your body's FAT programs.

Addressing the REAL Causes of Obesity

The Gabriel Method is therefore a way of losing weight by systematically dealing with the real causes of obesity.

By addressing and eliminating the real reasons your body wants to hold on to weight, you can switch your FAT programs off. Your body then, wants to be thinner and actually works with you and assists you in your weightloss effort. When your body wants to be thinner, you lose weight easily and naturally. You simply start to crave less food, you crave healthier food, your metabolism increases and you become very efficient at burning fat.

Food is just one small part of the equation. But when it comes to food, it's not about subtracting foods. It's about adding the foods that have the nutrients your body needs in a form that you can easily digest and assimilate.

One of the primary reasons our FAT programs get activated is that we are in a chronic state of nutritional starvation.

Most modern-day, man-made, conventionally-farmed and processed foods are nutritionally barren, devitalised and highly toxic. In addition, they cause digestive problems and it's the ensuing hormonal chaos and cellular stress that activate FAT programs. These man-made "fake" foods also cause erratic blood sugar fluctuations and junk food cravings.

Over time this toxic assault on our bodies depletes our immune systems, clogs our arteries, causes cellular breakdown and leads to chronic disease and conditions such as sleep apnea; type-2 diabetes, inflammation, chronic fatigue, heart disease, arthritis, food allergies, asthma, leaky gut syndrome, Crohn's disease and cancer.

Furthermore, poor nutrition from distressed and toxic food may be responsible for some forms of depression, bi-polar disease, ADD and autism. To add insult to injury, many of the medications we take as a response to these chronic diseases are, in themselves, toxic to the liver and can also activate the FAT programs, causing further weight gain in addition to all the other problems.

Losing weight, or to be more accurate, losing excess fat, is never simply about calories in and calories out, it's about choosing the highest quality, least toxic ingredients available; ingredients that are full of life-force vitality and essential nutrients. When you are properly nourished, your body will determine your best weight and how many calories your body requires. When your body wants to be thin, you will naturally want fewer calories.

Losing weight is not about low fat or low carbohydrates either. It's about healthy fats and healthy carbs. Healthy fat is one of the best things you can put in your body and unhealthy fat is one of the worst, and the same can be said for carbs. So learning how to replace bad fats with good fats, and bad carbs with good ones is a major factor in understanding how to nourish your body and how to turn the FAT programs off.

That's what our super-delicious, super-nutritious recipes are all about.

The beauty of these simple principles is that, with a little practice, you can quickly learn how to replace dead, toxic ingredients with fresh, live, vibrant, super-healthy ingredients and still make it taste just as amazing as so-called 'normal' food. Many of these recipes are the culmination of nearly 10 years of perfecting the art of super-delicious, super-nutritious cooking. You are definitely in for a treat!

I'd encourage you to have fun finding new super-healthy, live, vital, cost-effective foods wherever you can at your local supermarket, farmers markets, health food store and growing co-ops. Enjoy growing your own vegetables in a garden, and relish preparing these beautiful dishes for yourself and your family. Use them as a basis to create your own favourites, and please share your recipes with the ever growing Gabriel Method community. We'd love to hear from you!

Yours in Super Delicious Health!

Jon

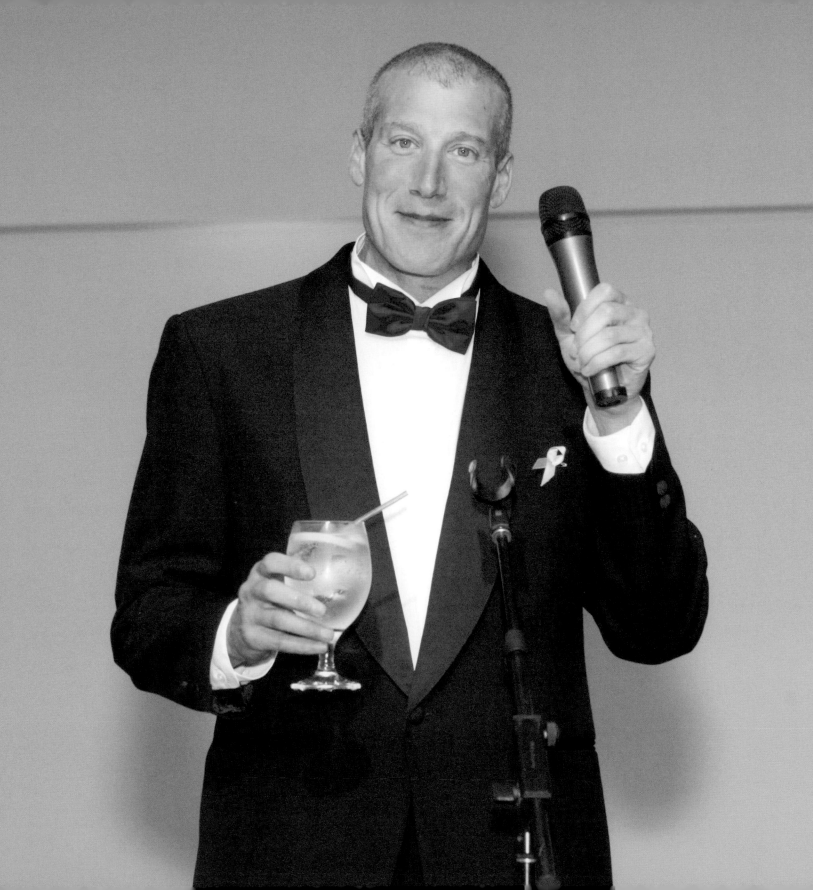

The Basics of Gabrielicious Eating!

Our recipes are designed to nourish and inspire. Our meals, snacks and desserts are super– delicious. They are also super-nutritious and will encourage better health and more effective weightloss.

In general, a proper Gabriel Method meal should have the three vital ingredients:

Omega-3 Fatty Acids
Protein
Live Food

Omega-3 fatty acids are found in cold water fish and fish oils and some nuts and seeds, particularly flax seeds (linseeds) and chia seeds.

Protein is found in meat, fish, eggs, dairy, nuts and seeds and some combinations of vegetables.

Live foods are fresh, unprocessed, uncooked, fruits and vegetables, in particular green leafy lettuce, sprouts and live, green juices.

The presence of these three factors nourishes your body, helps turn off your FAT programs and keeps your blood sugar levels stable for long periods of time. Unstable blood sugar means peaks and troughs; peaks that inhibit weightloss and troughs that cause junk food cravings, thus activating starvation signals and perpetuating the FAT programs.

Great things happen when your blood sugar levels remain stable: You have more energy and less hunger and you start living off of your fat reserves instead of the junk food industry living off you. This is where the transformation begins to really happen.

So ask yourself at every meal:
Where are the Omega-3s?
Where's the protein?
Where's the live food?

Remember to Keep the Focus on Adding

The Gabriel Method is about adding, rather than subtracting, foods. That's not to say however, that there aren't foods that we want to avoid, there are. But this Method is about turning your body on to the right foods without suffering from feelings of hunger or deprivation. It's about adding foods that make your body feel truly satiated, and naturally eliminating cravings for false foods.

Even if you're currently eating junk food, just add the good stuff where you can, and your body will start to tell you it wants the healthy alternatives and the cravings will subside. Incorporating our recipes into your weekly meal plan is a fantastic, easy and enjoyable way to start.

Please refer to chapters 9-15 of The Gabriel Method for more information about how adding protein, Omega-3s and live food can totally change your life. The more you know about what your food choices are doing (and not doing) for you, the better equipped you will be at integrating the Method into your life-style.

Gabrielising Your Meals

You can continue to indulge in whatever food you desire for as long as you want though we strongly recommend that you 'Gabrielise' your meals. Any meal, even take-away meals, can be Gabrielised by turning them into a salad and including live foods as well as protein and Omega-3 fatty acids. Chop up a hamburger, add salad greens and a high-quality dressing and you can effectively Gabrielise even one of the world's most popular fast foods.

You can also Gabrielise your favourite recipes by simple substitution. I totally understand that you love your grandmother's fabulous recipe for lasagne, but nothing is stopping you from using organic cheese and grass-fed ground beef and, instead of pasta strips, you can use strips of zucchini. OK, it won't be exactly the same but you might really like the result anyway.

The general principle is that if you're preparing a cold dish then use the healthy cold oils. These are the oils rich in Omega-3 fatty acids, like flax seed oil, chia seed oil and walnut oil. These oils are great when cold but you can't cook with them because the essential nutrients will be corrupted.

If you're preparing a hot dish, use healthy cooking oils, such as ghee, coconut oil and cold-pressed rice bran oil, as these oils can withstand heat. And if you're sweetening things up, use our recommended alternative natural sweeteners.

The following recipes are what we call 'Gabrielicious'. We hope you have as much fun and satisfaction in preparing them, and sharing them, as we have.

In most cases we have 'Gabrielised' our existing favourites. That is to say, we have taken our favourite foods and added Omega-3s, protein and live foods, used good cooking oils and substituted bad or toxic ingredients – such as 'dead carbs' and artificial ingredients – for better alternatives.

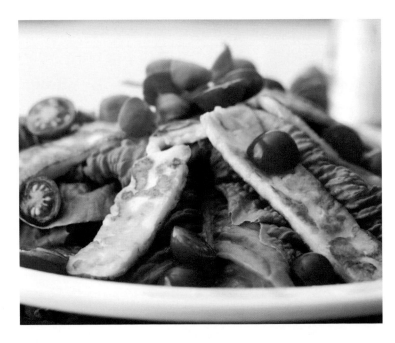

We hope you'll feel inspired and empowered to do the same, so we have added Gabrielising tips for adding and substituting, throughout the book, that will help you to customise this Method and transform your personal, favourite snacks and meals.

The Gabriel-Friendly Kitchen

Here's a list of some things that I have in my pantry and kitchen that are not so commonly used, or that might need to be purchased from a specialised health-food store. The condiments, vinegars, seasonings, sweeteners and oils, listed below, are all natural alternatives chosen for their nutritious and delicious properties.

Adding these items to your pantry will help you to incorporate our Gabrielicious recipes into your weekly meal planning.

Apple Cider Vinegar

Apple cider vinegar is a light brownish or yellow vinegar made from pulverised apples. It is regarded as an especially helpful health tonic, which can help conditions such as obesity and diabetes and improve digestion. You can use it on salad, or simply take two tablespoons a day in a glass of water.

Balsamic Vinegar

Balsamic vinegar is a rich, dark vinegar, whose sweet taste makes it very mellow and pleasant to use in salads and other dishes. Balsamic vinegar contains powerful antioxidants called polyphenols, which inhibit cell damage and boost the immune system. These antioxidants have the potential to protect against heart disease, cancer, and other inflammatory conditions.

Healthy Salt – Himalayan Salt Crystals, Celtic Salt, Sea Salt

Natural salts are loaded with trace minerals necessary for all cellular functions. Himalayan salt, in particular, comes from a region in Pakistan that is known for its highly mineral-dense salts. It is gray or even pinkish in color. Any "sea salt", or minimally processed salt, is a good substitute for table salt, and always look for a dirty grey color (this is natural). Try to avoid normal table salt as it's been bleached, over processed and highly toxic.

Tamari

This Japanese condiment is very similar to a classic soy sauce, but has a more robust and often sweeter flavour. It's a healthy substitute for salt, as eating too much salt can lead to high blood pressure which can lead to a heart attack or stroke. If you don't have tamari, you can use an organic soy sauce instead. It's a great addition to stir fries and other vegetable or meat dishes.

Chia Seeds

Chia is a plant which, like flaxseed, has a great deal of healthy Omega-3 fatty acid in it. Omega-3 fatty acids are anti-inflammatory, essential for the health of your brain, and they give you sustained energy throughout the day. You can find chia seeds at most health food stores, and you can add them to salads, cereals or smoothies.

Whole Flax Seeds (Linseeds)

These nutritious seeds have a subtle, nutty flavour and are packed with Omega-3 fatty acids and dietary fibre. Always buy flax seeds in their whole seed form (not ground) and store them in the refrigerator. Once you grind the seed the essential oil begins to go rancid. So grind them just prior to use in a coffee grinder.

Maca Powder

Maca is a world-renown revitalising superfood that is used by both men and women seeking a natural boost in energy, hormonal balance and vitality. It is created by grinding the root of the Peruvian maca plant, and is taken as a supplement, or can be used in several dishes. It helps the body to regulate hormonal processes and increases blood circulation in your body. Because of its ability to stabilise hormones, maca can also support emotional healing.

Nori Sheets

Perhaps the most well known seaweed, Nori is used to make sushi in Japanese restaurants and is sold in most supermarkets and health food stores in dry sheets that are very easy to use as wraps, or chopped and sprinkled on any savoury dish. Seaweed, in general, is packed full of much needed vitamins and minerals, including some relatively rare trace elements. Nori is rich in calcium iodine and iron and quite high in protein. It is also a good source of Vitamin C, Vitamin A, potassium, magnesium and riboflavin (B2). Not only does it have all these nutritional riches, it is also a low-fat food.

Miso Paste

Made from soybeans, miso is a natural fermented product with many nutritional benefits. With considerable quantities of trace minerals such as manganese, zinc and copper, this great tasting paste can be used as a soup to enhance the flavour of meat and vegetable dishes.

Almonds

Almonds are high in monounsaturated fats, the same type of health promoting fats as are found in olive oil, which have been associated with reduced risk of heart disease. They also have high amounts of Vitamin E, which is great for your skin and your immune system.

Hazelnuts

Hazelnuts are an excellent source of polyunsaturated and monounsaturated fats that help to protect heart health. They're also high in protein and fibre. A cup of chopped hazelnuts has a whopping 17 grams of protein and 11 grams of fibre. Hazelnuts are an excellent source of Vitamin E as well as the B Vitamins including folate. They're also a good source of potassium, calcium, and magnesium which help to maintain a healthy blood pressure.

Walnuts

Walnuts are one of the best plant sources of protein. They are rich in fibre, B Vitamins, magnesium, and antioxidants such as Vitamin E. They're a great snack option and can be used in salads too.

Pumpkin Seeds (Pepitas)

Pumpkin seeds, also known as pepitas, are flat, dark green seeds that are extremely nutritious and flavourful. Pepitas are particularly good for bone strength, and have an anti-inflammatory effect which can help in easing the pain of arthritis. They also provide a wide range of traditional nutrients, such as minerals, protein and monounsaturated fat, making them a nutritious and guilt-free snack.

Sesame Seeds

Sesame seeds add a nutty taste and a delicate, almost invisible, crunch to many Asian dishes and salads. They are extremely rich in beneficial minerals and can help boost vascular and respiratory health, as well as lower cholesterol.

Spirulina

Spirulina is a fresh water algae which is incredibly high in protein as well as minerals and vitamins. It has an amazing list of health benefits including boosting the immune system, improving digestion, reducing fatigue, boosting energy levels and it helps to control appetite. It is usually taken as a supplement, but can be used in recipes as well.

Tahini

Tahini is a thick paste made from ground sesame seeds. Originating from the Middle East, tahini is full of nutrients some of which include, iron, manganese, calcium and zinc. We use it in a variety of recipes in this book.

Unsweetened Cocoa Powder

When people think of chocolate as unhealthy, they are referring more to the commercially over processed, refined chocolate we find on supermarket shelves. However, cocoa, the component in its raw form, is filled with antioxidants and many health-boosting minerals. Interestingly, cocoa has more antioxidants than any other food, including blueberries, red wine, and black and green teas. Unsweetened, raw cocoa powder is actually a supremely healthy food that can be used in baking and to make hot chocolate.

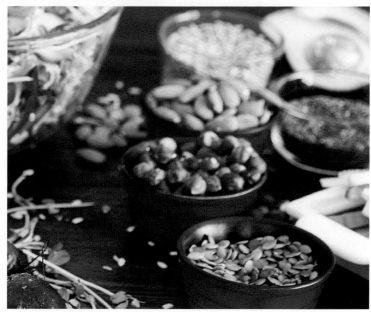

Coconut Flour

Coconut flour is healthy and delicious. High in protein and dietary fibre, it is gluten-free and hypoallergenic. We find it works really well when combined with eggs as in our Blueberry Ricotta Pancakes (see page 42).

Unsweetened, Unflavoured Whey Protein Concentrate

Preferably from grass-fed cows, goat's or sheep's milk. Whey Protein Concentrate is a very assimilable source of protein. As it has no distinct taste or flavour, it can be easily incorporated into drinks, desserts and other liquid or creamy recipes.

Refrigerated Items

Frozen Berries, Frozen Bananas and Other Fruit

It's a great idea to keep some fruit in your freezer, to have it on hand for making smoothies and other healthy snacks. Berries, in particular, are packed with antioxidants and bananas are a great source of energy for that midday lull.

Grass-Fed Meats, Free Range Chicken and Free Range Eggs

Whenever possible, try to buy your meat, chicken and eggs from local farmers and ideally farmers who raise their animals according to organic, grass-fed, and free range standards. Naturally raised animals are much more nutritious.

Also, try to find Omega-3 enriched eggs, as these will give you an extra boost to your immune system.

Wild, Fresh Fish

Fish farming is a fast-growing industry, and while it may seem harmless enough, it has been discovered that farmed fish contains many more contaminants, such as pesticides and antibiotics, than fresh fish. Farmed fish are also generally less nutritious than wild fish. They tend to have less protein and less Omega-3 fats than their wild counterparts.

Plain Organic Yoghurt – preferably from goat's or sheep's milk

Organic yoghurt is a great source of the 'good bacteria', or probiotics, that we require to keep our digestive systems healthy. These probiotics provide their benefits by adjusting the microflora (the natural balance of organisms) in the intestines, and by boosting digestion and immune function. When shopping, keep in mind that the only yoghurts that contain probiotics are those that say "live and active cultures" on the label.

Nut Milk

Too much dairy can cause inflammation, which activates the FAT Programs. Cheese and yoghurt are not as bad because they have no lactose or milk sugar. So, while we still use cheese and yoghurt in many of our recipes, we are always looking for suitable replacements for drinking milk.

For this reason, we recommend using nut milk instead. Nut milk is made from soaking and grinding nuts and seeds like almonds, hazelnuts and sunflower seeds. It tastes great and has all the benefits of protein and essential fats that nuts and seeds provide, without sacrificing taste.

You can use it as a substitute for milk in cereals, smoothies and ice creams. It is very easy to make (see page 256) and more cost effective than buying it.

Gabrielicious Cold Oils

Use these oils for salad dressings, smoothies and other cold Gabrilicious recipes.

Flaxseed (Linseed) Oil

Flax seeds, also known as linseeds, are very high in Omega-3 fatty acids and are beneficial to nearly every system in our body, such as the nervous system, cardiovascular system, reproductive system, immune system, and circulatory system. The natural properties of flaxseed oil offer hundreds of health benefits, such as helping with skin problems, lowering high blood pressure and cholesterol, fighting obesity and improving the immune system. You can drizzle flaxseed oil over your salads or use it in your salad dressing. It doesn't respond well to heat, so don't use it for cooking.

Chia seed Oil

Chia seed oil is also extremely high in Omega-3s, antioxidants and minerals, making it especially beneficial for your immune system. It's usually sold as capsules, which should be kept refrigerated, but can sometimes be found as a regular oil which you can use to dress your salads.

Walnut Oil

Walnut oil, another good source of Omega-3 fatty acids, is quite difficult to find, mainly because it's more expensive and has a shorter shelf life than most oils. It is popular though as it has a very nutty flavour which gives a great edge to salads and other ready-cooked dishes.

*Note: All of the above oils should always be refrigerated and used within 4 months of manufacturing.

Organic Extra Virgin Olive Oil

Olive oil is not high in Omega-3 fatty acids but it's high in other essential fats. It also has a much more mild taste that the other cold oils we recommend. For this reason, we use it in most of our salad dressings.

'Gabriel Friendly Cooking Oils'

Heat corrupts most oils, especially those high in essential fatty acids. Once corrupted, the oil becomes highly toxic. So when you're frying, choose oils that are more resistant to high temperatures. The following oils are more resistant to higher temperatures, and make for ideal cooking oils.

Ghee

Ghee is "cooked down" or "clarified" butter, and because it's been clarified, it's considered to have fewer impurities than regular butter. It's a traditional cooking fat in Indian cuisine (it's a very stable fat and can be heated) and has a rich flavour that goes with just about anything. It can be used instead of butter, and many people believe it has health benefits such as boosting your immune system and enhancing digestion.

Cold Pressed Rice Bran Oil

Rice bran oil is the oil extracted from the germ and inner husk of rice. It has a mild flavour and is great to use in high-temperature cooking methods such as stir-frying and deep-frying. It is considered a heart-healthy oil as it helps to lower cholesterol levels. It is also high in Vitamin E, which is great for your skin, as well as being a powerful antioxidant.

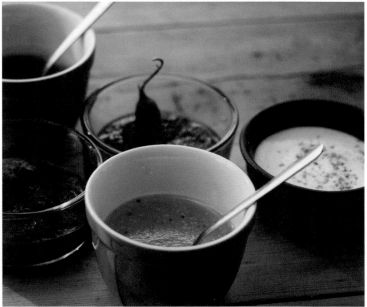

Avocado Oil

Avocado oil is pressed from the fruit of the avocado, and has a host of health benefits compared with other oils. It's very heat tolerant, making it a great oil to cook with. It's also a heart-healthy oil that won't encourage weight gain or changes in your cholesterol or blood pressure levels.

Coconut Oil

Coconut oil is made from pressing coconuts, and it's been used in traditional tropical cultures for thousands of years. It's a great option for cooking, as it's heat-resistant, and it also has heaps of health benefits. It promotes heart health, promotes weight loss, boosts your immune system and supports a healthy metabolism. It's also great for your skin, leaving it healthy and youthful looking.

*Note: All Gabrielicious oil should be 'cold pressed', not refined. The beneficial qualities of the oils get destroyed in the refining process.

Gabrielicious Sweeteners

Getting a Little Healthy Sweetness Into Your Life

Here at The Gabriel Method, we are nothing if not realists. We know that when your FAT programs are on, your sense of sweetness is diminished, so you're therefore going to crave increasingly higher sugar-content foods.

Getting Super Delicious / Super Nutritous sweeteners is an art in itself. Most common, refined table sugars and syrups spike your insulin levels and lead to a condition known as hyper-insulinemia or "perpetually elevated insulin levels". Insulin is the principal fat storage hormone and when your insulin levels are elevated your body goes into perpetual fat storage mode.

What's worse is, that when you have elevated insulin levels you actually lose the ability to burn fat. You also lose the ability to regulate your blood sugar, leading to sudden, low blood sugar episodes that cause ravenous junk food cravings. So the more sugar you eat, the more you crave.

It's a vicious cycle and, for this reason and many others, it's important to find a suitable alternative. What is a suitable alternative to sugar? One that tastes great but doesn't elevate your insulin levels. Artificial sweeteners are definitely out as they can activate your FAT programs too. This is a perfect example of how it's not just about calories in and calories out.

Artificial sweeteners have zero calories but contain toxic chemicals that trigger your brain to turn on the FAT programs. Sure, your calorie intake may be lower, but over time you are hungrier, craving more fattening foods; your metabolism slows down so you become tired all the time and burn fewer calories, making your body even less able to lose excess fat.

Artificial sweeteners also cause many other health problems, including depression, bi-polar disease and digestion problems. So we need a natural sweetener that tastes good but doesn't elevate your blood sugar and insulin levels.

The solution? A combination of natural sweeteners.

Unfortunately no one sweetener fits the bill at the moment, but we've worked with a combination of them that work well under different circumstances.

Natural Sweeteners

Stevia

Stevia is a South American herb whose leaves are ground to make a natural sweetener. Stevia can be as much as 200 times sweeter than table sugar, so just a pinch is equivalent to one or two tablespoons of sugar. It has zero calories and does not elevate blood sugar levels though it does have a slightly bitter aftertaste, so we've found Stevia works best with fruits and foods that are slightly tart. It brings out the naturally occurring sweetness nicely, but with chocolate and other bitter things, it isn't nearly as effective. In fact it can bring out the bitterness even more.

Xylitol

Xylitol is also a natural sweetener derived from various fruits and vegetables but you can also find it in mushrooms, oats, birch bark and even corn husks. It's about the same sweetness as sugar but has only two-thirds the calories. It barely elevates your blood sugar, registering 7 on the glycemic index, as compared to 65 or 70 with table sugar. Xylitol tastes great, you can cook with it, it has no bitter aftertaste and it even helps your body to absorb calcium. However, xylitol is processed, so it's not super healthy, and if you have too much of it, it can cause digestion problems like excess gas. We recommend using xylitol sparingly.

Coconut Palm Sugar

I love almost everything about this sweetener. It's natural, easy to digest, has a beautiful, caramel, sweet taste, but it elevates your blood sugar a bit higher than xylitol and stevia. It's about a 35 on the GI. Not too bad, but still bad enough that it can cause problems in large doses and in susceptible people.

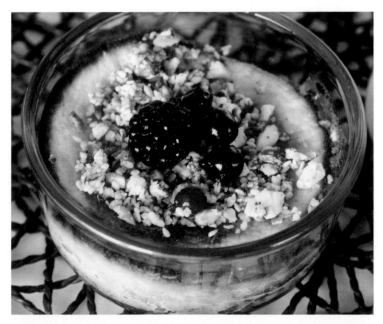

In the recipes in this book you'll see that we use different combinations of these three sweeteners, depending on the recipe.

As a general rule though you can combine all three sweeteners to get the best of all worlds. We're currently perfecting a Gabriel Method proprietary sweetener that uses these three in a specific combination.

But for now try this as an all-purpose sugar substitute natural sweetener:

1 Tablespoon Xylitol
1 Tablespoon Organic Coconut Palm Sugars
A pinch of Stevia

This combination tastes great and doesn't elevate your blood sugar too much. You can cook with it, bake with it and there's no bitter aftertaste.

In all the recipes that require a sweetener, you can use the sweeteners suggested or you can use this special blend that we've formulated. It's up to you. Either way you'll be getting a great treat!

Supplements

Digestive Enzymes

Digestive enzymes are molecules that help to break down the food in the body so that the nutrients can be absorbed. Raw live foods are a great source of digestive enzymes. They can also be taken in supplement form.

Probiotics

These are living micro-organisms found in the gut that have a healthy effect on your digestion. They are common in fermented foods such as yoghurt, soy yoghurt and kefir (must be unpasteurised).

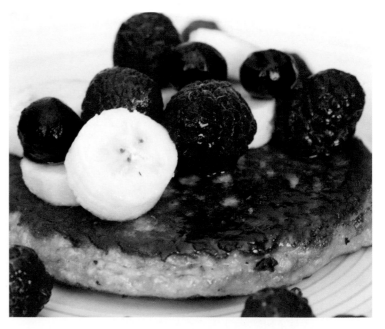

Tools

Coffee Grinder or Mortar and Pestle

It is best to crush most seeds and spices as you use them, as they can otherwise go rancid, or lose their nutritional value, especially flax seeds. It's useful to have an electric coffee grinder or mortar and pestle to do so.

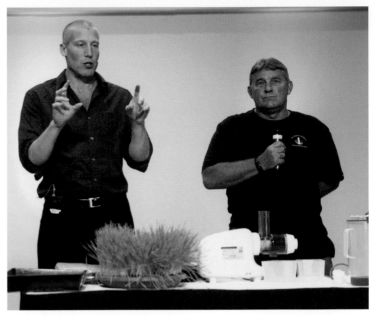

Food Processor

A food processor is an electric kitchen appliance used for chopping, mixing, or puréeing foods. It is useful for making soups, smoothies and sauces, or for chopping up vegetables for a variety of dishes.

Hand-Held Stick Blender

Also known as a bar mix or hand-held blender, the stick blender is particularly useful for making smoothies and dessert recipes.

Slow Masticating Juicer

Masticating juicers are extremely versatile juicers, as they use a two-step process to extract more juice from your fruit or vegetables. They come in 1 or 2-auger versions, and the slow moving auger literally "chews" the juice out of plants. Aside from making great juices, they also make wonderful nut butters and sorbets.

Dehydrator

A dehydrator is a special appliance that removes moisture from food in order to preserve it. It's very popular in the raw food movement as it enables you to make healthy versions of crackers, breads, cookies and many other things. Raw foodies dehydrate their foods at temperatures below 40°C / 105°F so that the nutrients remain intact and do not get corrupted or destroyed, as they would do at higher temperatures.

Organic Foods

There is a lot of ongoing debate about organic foods versus conventional foods. The Gabriel Method is unreservedly on the side of organic foods, even though they are currently more expensive than non-organic. However buying non-organic to save money is really the most false of false economies.

Non-organic foods can have up to 20 different pesticides, herbicides, fungicides and other toxic chemicals used in their production. These chemicals are totally foreign to our bodies. When faced with many of these toxins, our bodies often have no other way to respond other than to store them in fat cells.

The most cutting edge research now points to toxins as a major source of stress that activates our FAT programs. Turning on the FAT programs means that you will be hungrier and eat more, so on balance, your overall food bill will increase.

The accumulation of poisons in your system can cause disease and ill-health. Should I also mention that all this sickness will need medication which is costly and also toxic? So when you look at the big picture, organic makes sense at every level-physical, mental, emotional, energetic and financial.

That being said, there are many cheaper alternatives to organic. Visit your regional farmers markets and growing co-ops and you'll find locally grown, in season, spray-free produce and grass fed meats and dairy. Most of the produce is even cheaper than what you would find at a supermarket because there's no middleman. Also, locally grown means it will be much fresher and have more life force vitality than organic foods that have been shipped thousands of miles. It's really a question of being creative and expanding your awareness. And that's exactly what our recipes are all about. So let's get into it and start enjoying the good stuff!

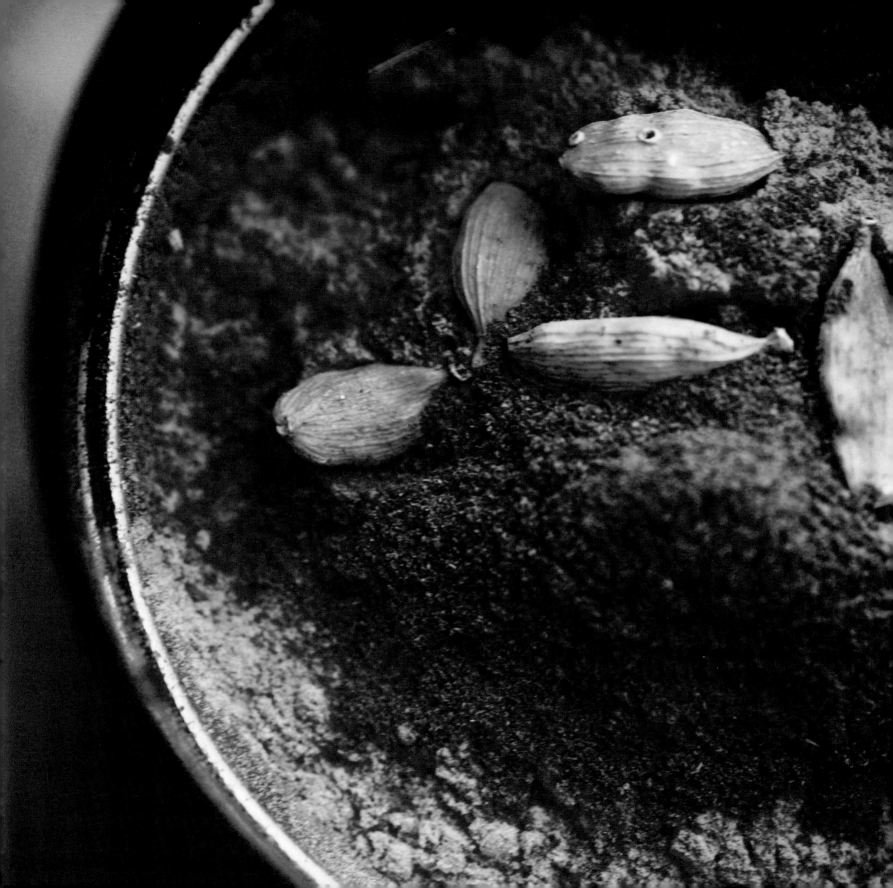

Breakfast

It's a cliché, but nevertheless true, that breakfast is the most important meal of the day. As far as The Gabriel Method is concerned, breakfast is especially important for the following reasons;

A good, full breakfast will:

- Replenish you after the fasting hours of sleep.

- Stabilise your blood sugar so that you don't get cravings for junk food in the late mornings and afternoons.

- Give you more energy to kickstart your day, and because you have more energy you'll feel less stressed.

- Help turn off the FAT programs because your body will feel properly nourished.

ANY RECIPE IN THIS BOOK CAN BE A BREAKFAST

It all depends on your inclination. The important thing to remember is that breakfast should include ALL of the big three: Omega-3 fatty acids, high-quality, assimilable protein and live, fresh foods filled with vitality. A vital breakfast is the key to a vital day.

In the following pages you will find a selection of meals that lend themselves to satisfying, hearty breakfasts although of course you can have any of these dishes whenever you want.

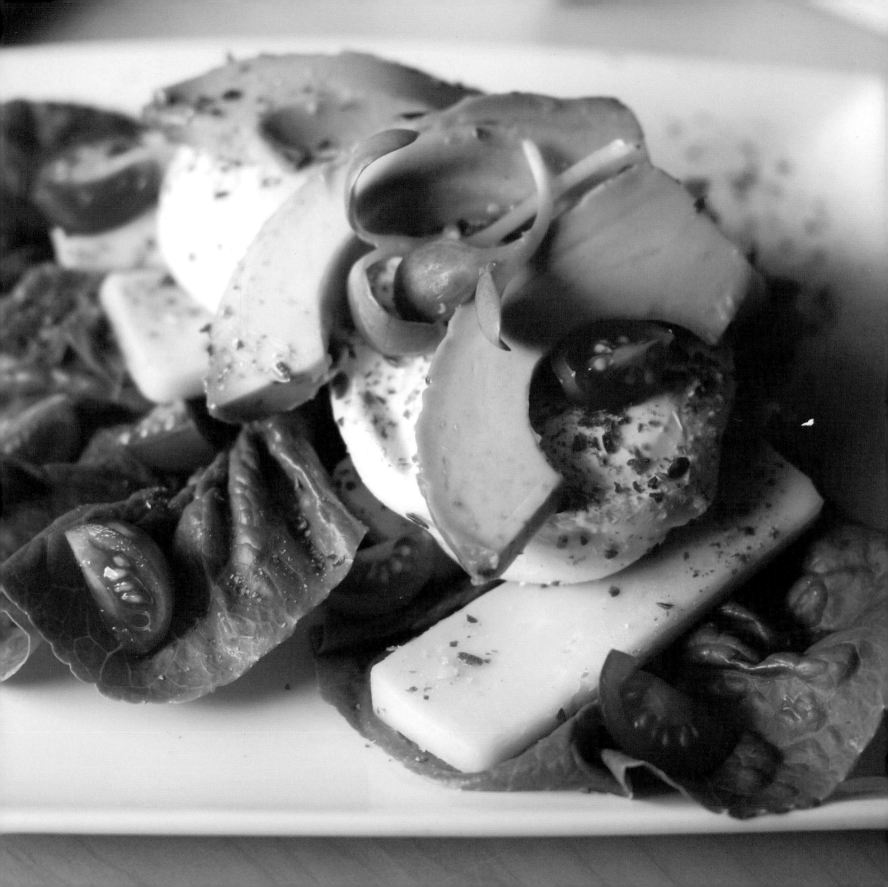

Breakfast

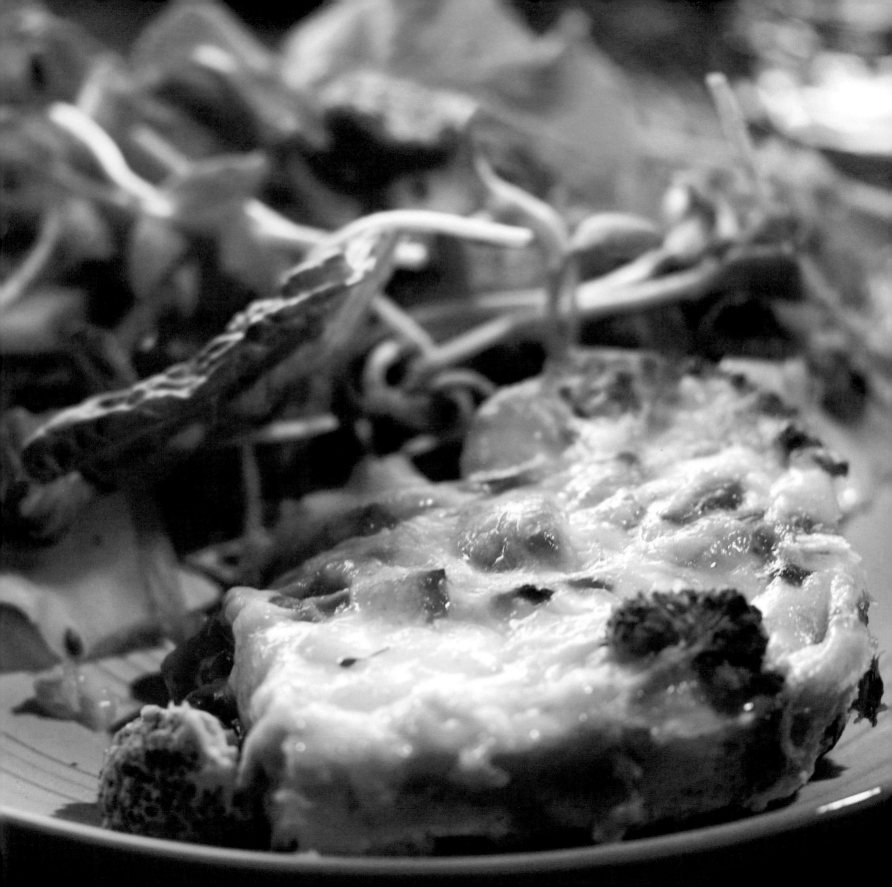

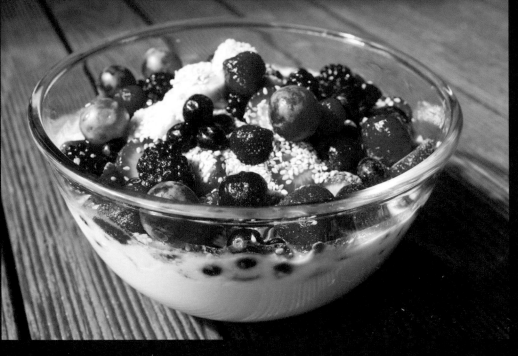

Jonny Chow

Serves: 1
Preparation time: 5 minutes

Ingredients:
½ cup organic plain yoghurt or
almond milk (see page 256)
30g natural whey protein powder
(unflavoured and unsweetened)
1 cup fresh fruit of choice*
1 tbsp ground flax seeds

Optional Extras:
Seeds such as sesame, chia, poppy, pumpkin.
xylitol or stevia for a sweetener
organic cocoa powder, unsweetened
cinnamon

*We like to use apple, bananas and berries though feel free to chop and change using seasonally available fresh fruit.

Method:
Mix all the ingredients together in a large bowl. Voilà! Savour the goodness.

This tasty recipe is affectionately named Jonny Chow by my friends because I so frequently have it for breakfast. I've made this breakfast for tens of thousands of people all over the world. If you've ever attended a Gabriel Method Seminar you would have shared this with me.

The principles are simple: we're using protein powder for our protein, flax or chia seeds for our Omega-3s and fresh seasonal fruit for our live food component to make this thick, nutty muesli-style breakfast. You can mix and match as you desire.

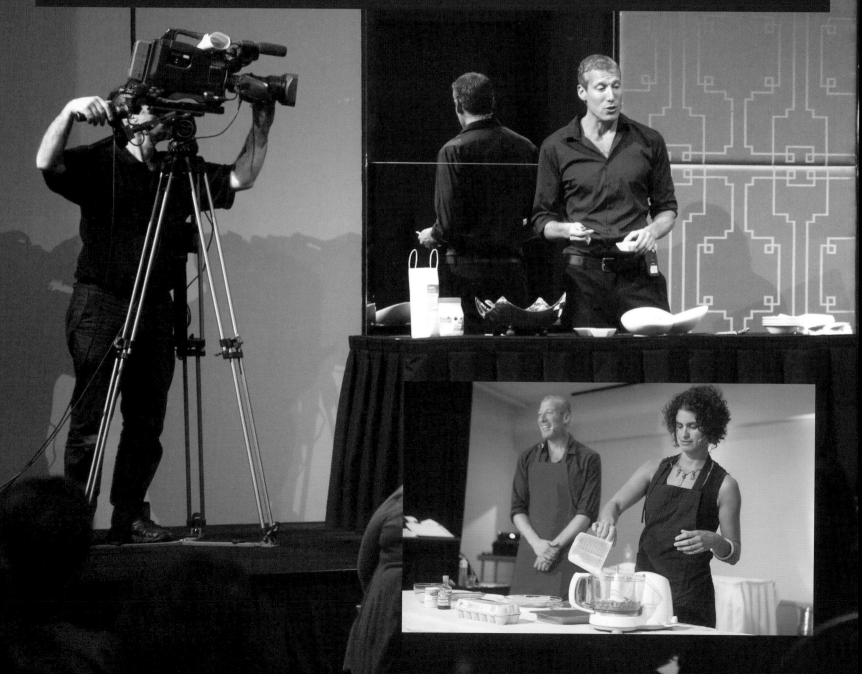

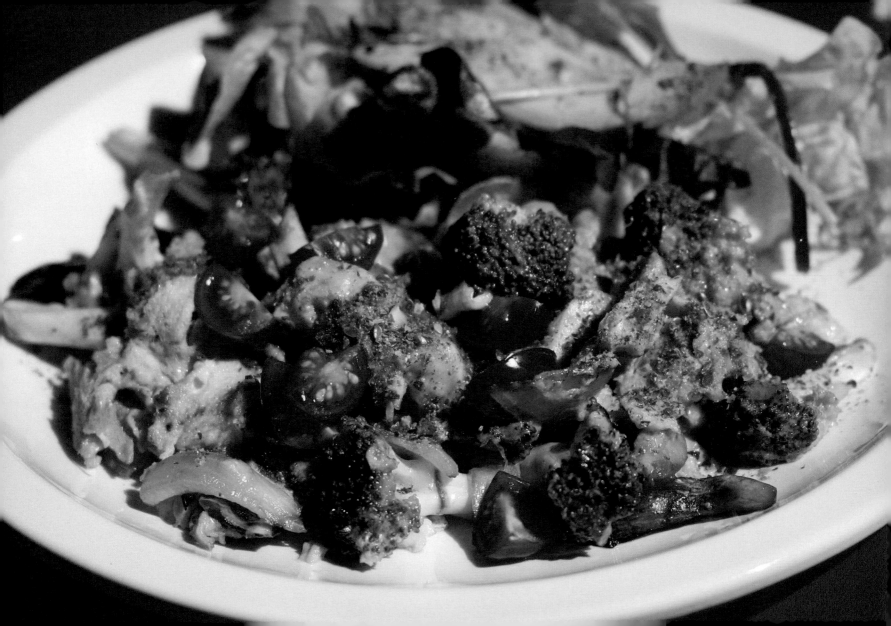

Scrambled Eggs

Serves: 2
Preparation time: 15 minutes
Cooking time: 10 minutes

Ingredients:

1 Tbsp ghee
1 brown onion, diced
1 cup broccoli, chopped
1 clove garlic, peeled and crushed

1 Tbsp tamari
4 eggs (organic, free range), beaten
¼ cup cheddar cheese, grated

Method:

1. Heat ghee in a frying pan on medium to high heat.
2. Add onion to pan and cook for a couple of minutes.
3. Reduce heat to medium and add broccoli, garlic and tamari. Cook while stirring for another minute or two.
4. Add beaten eggs to pan. Fold eggs and pan contents together until eggs are cooked. Add cheese and stir through until melted.
5. Serve sprinkled with ground flax seeds and a fresh salad!

"Scrambled eggs are a perfect way to please the whole family while using the ingredients in your fridge. Half a zucchini, those last few cherry tomatoes... throw it all in to this easy to prepare, and easier to enjoy meal."

Gabriel Method Breakfast Muesli

Serves: 8
Preparation time: 10 minutes
Serving size: ½ cup

Ingredients:

1½ cups almonds
⅓ cup pumpkin seeds
¾ cup sunflower seeds
¼ cup sesame seeds
¾ cup desiccated coconut
1 cup flax seeds

¼ cup almond butter
⅓ cup tahini
¼ cup coconut palm sugar
¼ cup water

Method:

1. Place all ingredients in food processor. Mix together until well combined and beginning to stick together.
2. Refrigerate mixture in airtight container. Serve with fresh fruit and nut milk as a delicious start to your day.

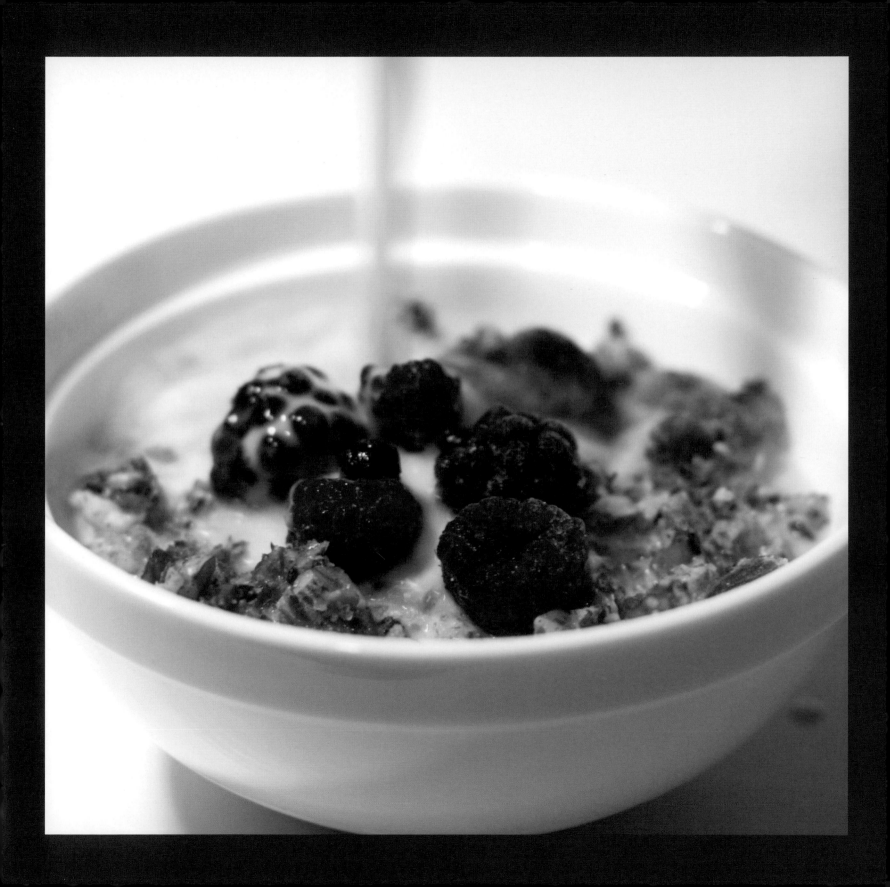

Blueberry Ricotta Pancakes

Makes: 6
Preparation time: 10 minutes
Cooking time: 10 minutes

Ingredients:
4 eggs (organic, free range)
100g ricotta cheese
¼ cup coconut flour
¼ cup chia seeds
1½ tsp coconut palm sugar or 1 tsp xylitol
½ cup blue berries, fresh or frozen

Method:
1. Whisk all ingredients, except blueberries, together thoroughly.
2. Add blueberries and gently stir through.
3. Pre heat pan on medium heat. Grease lightly with ghee or healthy cooking oil.
4. Put ¼ cup batter on pan, flatten out to about 1 cm thick. Brown on both sides.
5. It's finished when it's crispy on the outside but still a bit runny on the inside. Allow the middle to be slightly liquid. This way, the essential Omega-3 oil in the chia seeds will still remain mostly intact and the absorbant quality of the chia seeds will dry up the inside in a few minutes.
6. Serve with fresh fruit.

This is a great healthy way to get delicious pancakes that are loaded with proteins and Omega-3s without all the baddies.

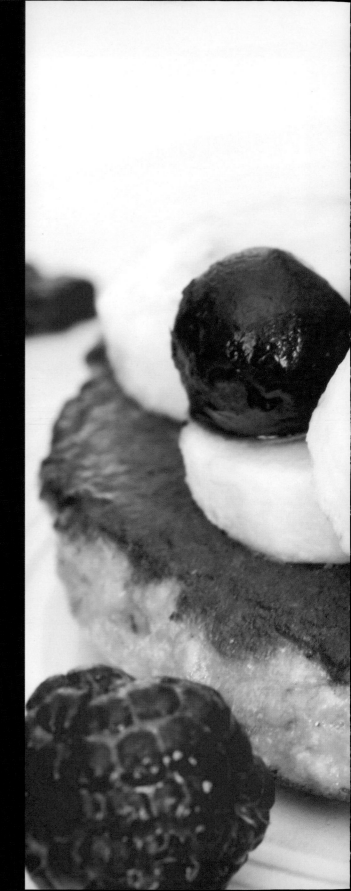

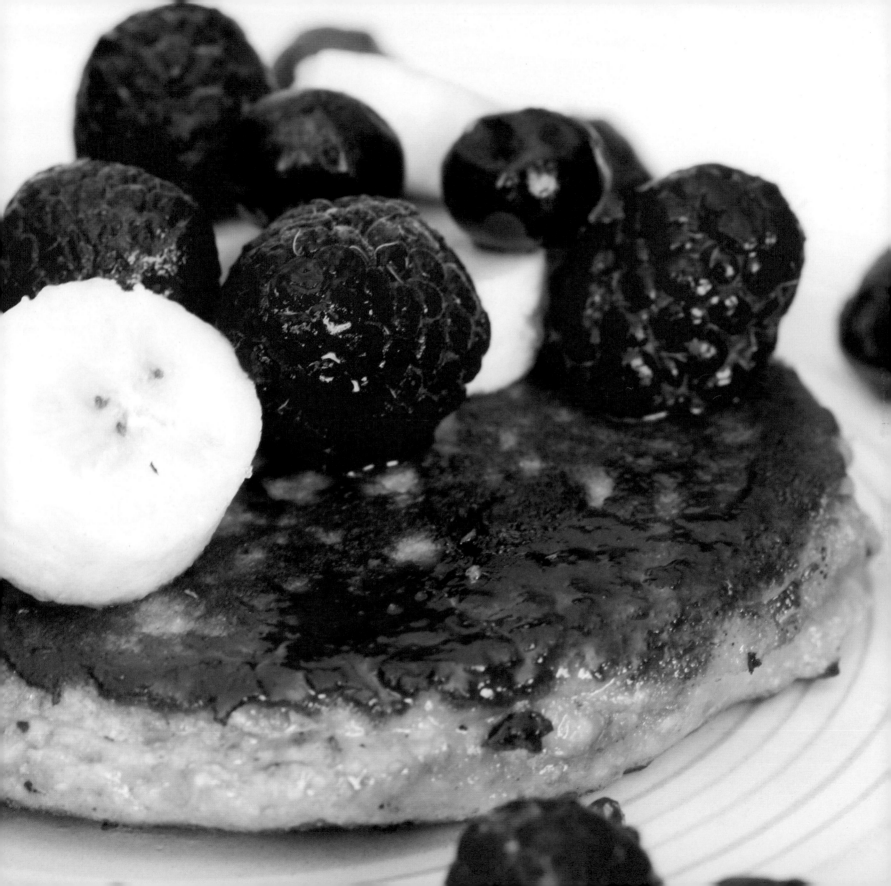

Poached Eggs with Havarti and Avocado

Serves: 1
Preparation time: 10 minutes
Cooking time: 3 minutes

Ingredients:
¼ cup vinegar
2 eggs (organic, free range)
2-3 lettuce leaves
35g havarti cheese
¼ avocado, sliced
1 Tbsp ground flax seeds

Method:
1. Fill medium saucepan halfway with water. Place on stove on high heat. Cover and leave to boil.
2. Place lettuce and havarti on plate. Slice avocado.
3. Once water is boiling, reduce heat to simmer. Add vinegar to water and stir water to create whirlpool. Crack eggs and slowly lower into spinning water.
4. Cook for 1 minute if you prefer a runny yolk or 2 minutes if you prefer a more solid yolk.
5. Scoop eggs out of saucepan using a slotted spoon and place them on top of lettuce and havarti. Place sliced avocado over eggs. Sprinkle with ground flax seeds.

"Poaching is one of the best ways to cook eggs as you preserve a larger percentage of healthy fat. This is one of our favourite lazy morning breakfasts."

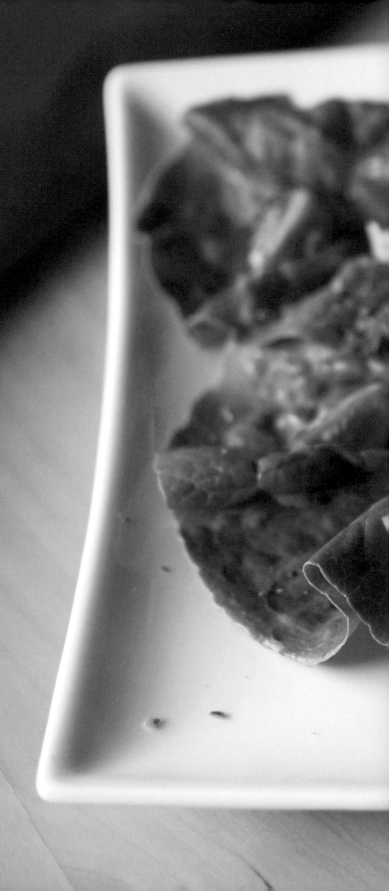

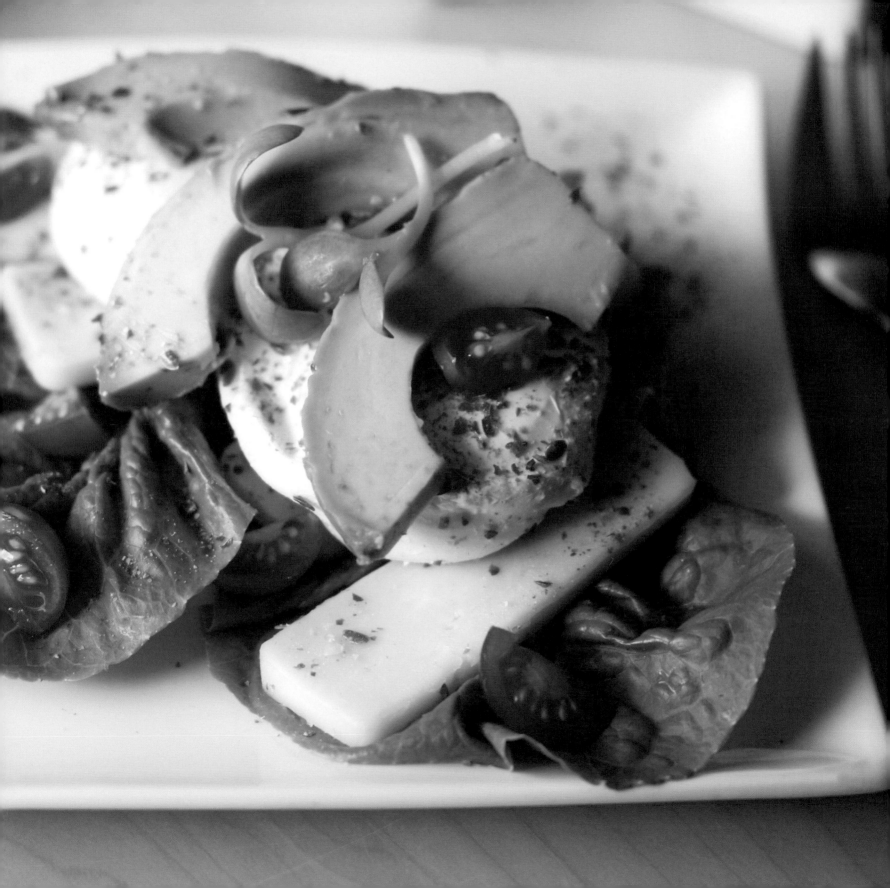

Poached Eggs with Smoked Salmon and Baby Spinach

Serves: 1
Preparation time: 10 minutes
Cooking time: 3 minutes

Ingredients:
¼ cup vinegar
2 eggs (organic, free range)
handful baby spinach leaves
50g smoked salmon
1 Tbsp ground flax seeds

Method:
1. Fill medium saucepan half way with water. Place on stove on high heat. Cover and leave to boil.
2. Place baby spinach leaves on plate, topped with smoked salmon.
3. Once water is boiling, reduce heat to simmer. Add vinegar to water and stir water to create whirlpool. Crack eggs and slowly lower into spinning water.
4. Cook for 1 minute if you prefer a runny yolk or 2 minutes if you prefer a more solid yolk.
5. Scoop eggs out of saucepan using a slotted spoon and place them on top of spinach and smoked salmon. Sprinkle with ground flax seeds and enjoy this fresh start to the day.

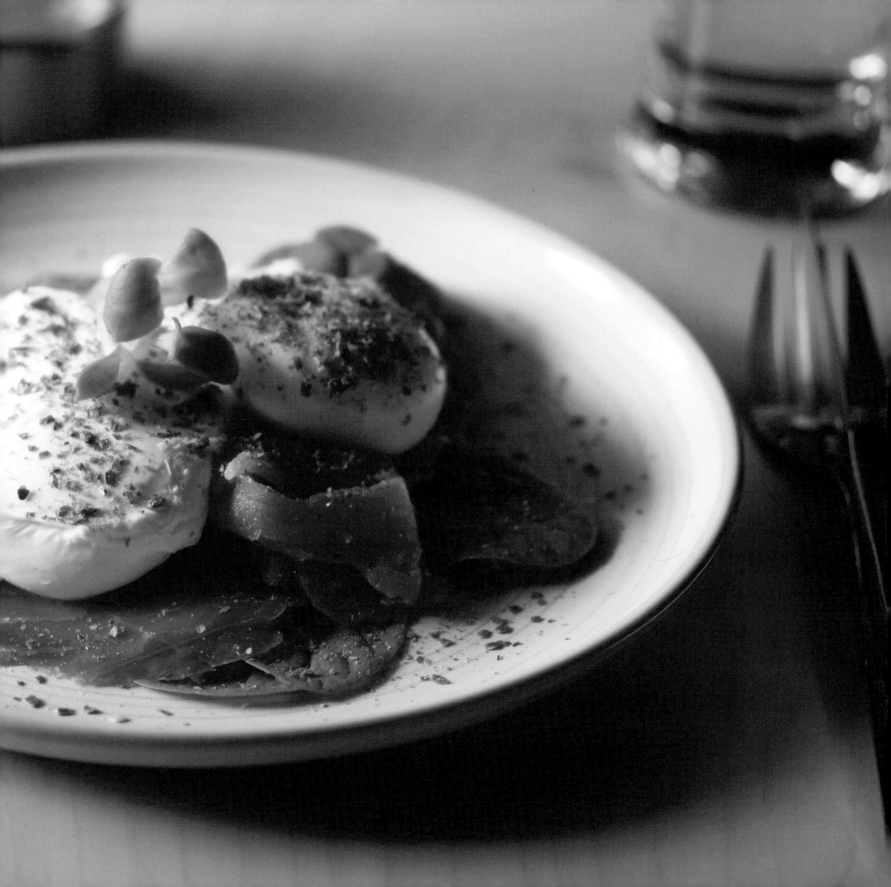

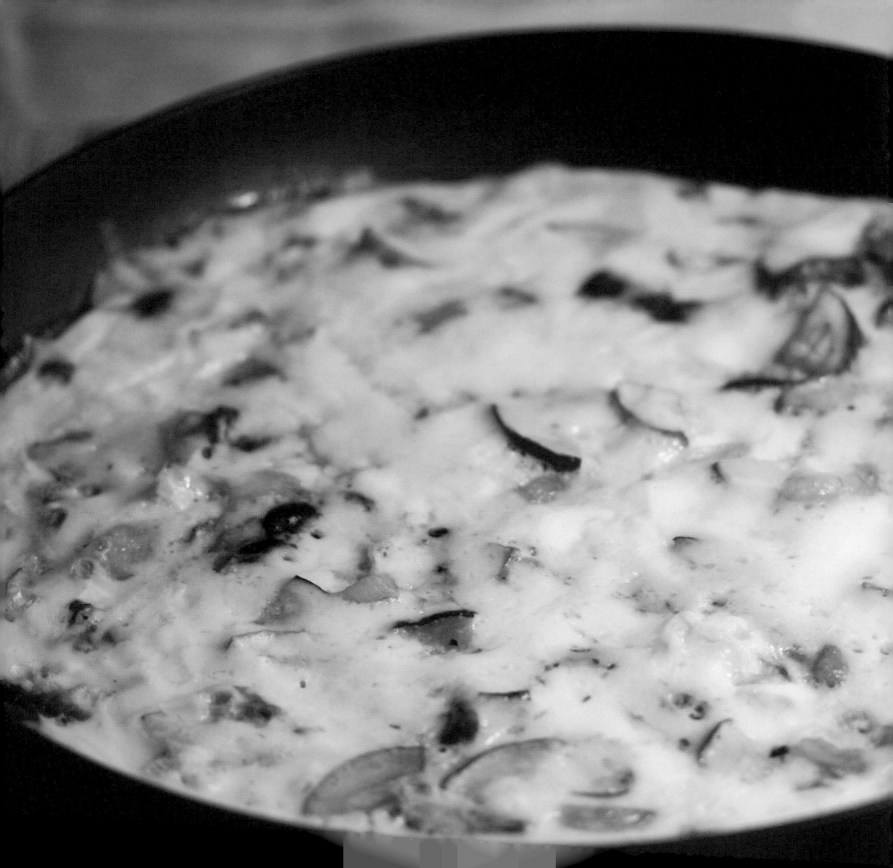

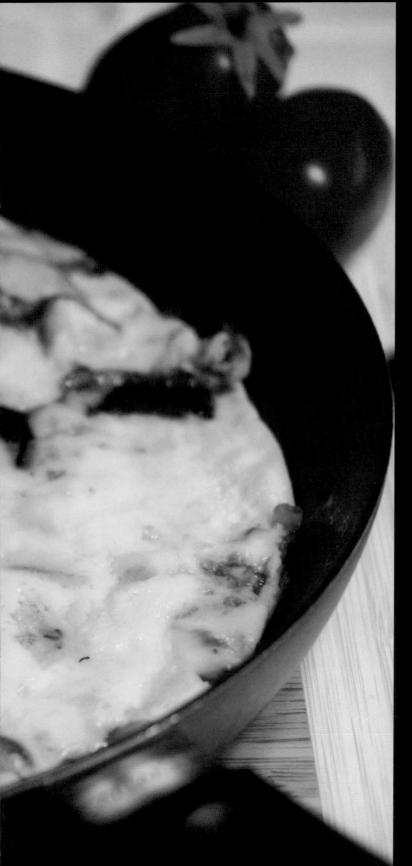

Zucchini and Mushroom Omelette

Serves: 4
Preparation time: 10 minutes
Cooking time: 20 minutes

Ingredients:
1 Tbsp ghee or Gabriel Method friendly oil (see page 24)
1 onion, sliced
½ zucchini, sliced and quartered
4 mushrooms, sliced
1 clove garlic, crushed
1 Tbsp tamari
6 eggs (organic, free range) beaten
35g cheese, grated

Method:
1. Melt ghee in frying pan on medium-high heat.
2. Place onion in frying pan and cook until slightly browned.
3. Add zucchini to pan as well as mushrooms, garlic and tamari. Cook while stirring for approximately 2 minutes. Beat eggs together.
4. Pour beaten eggs into frying pan over zucchini, mushroom mix.
5. Reduce heat to low. Cook for 3 minutes or until you can see that underside is cooked. Sprinkle cheese on top of omelette and cook covered for another minute or so until cheese has melted.

Frittatas - 3 different tastes

Serves: 6 for entree, 4 for main
Preparation time: 20 minutes
Cooking time: 45 minutes

Frittatas are a healthy and tasty way to get all your protein and greens without the dead carbs you get in a quiche. You can modify the basic frittata recipe by adding your favourite ingredients.

Broccoli & Red Capsicum (bell pepper) Frittata

Ingredients:

1 Tbsp ghee or Gabriel Method friendly cooking oil (see page 24)
1 onion
6 mushrooms, sliced
1 cup broccoli florets, sliced
½ cup red capsicum (bell pepper), sliced

1 clove garlic, crushed
1 Tbsp tamari
8 eggs (organic, free range), beaten
¼ cup tasty cheese, grated

Method:

1. Preheat oven to 180°C / 355°F. Grease 20cm square baking dish, lining the base with baking paper.
2. Heat cooking oil in frying pan over medium-high heat.
3. Add onion and cook until it begins to colour.
4. Add mushrooms, broccoli and red capsicum (bell pepper). Stir together, reducing to a medium heat. Add garlic and tamari. Stir to combine and allow to cook for another 2-3 minutes.
5. Beat the 8 eggs together in a medium bowl.
6. Transfer vegetables from frying pan to baking dish. Distribute well in the dish then pour beaten eggs over the top. Sprinkle the grated cheese on top.
7. Cook in oven for 35 minutes or until cooked through.

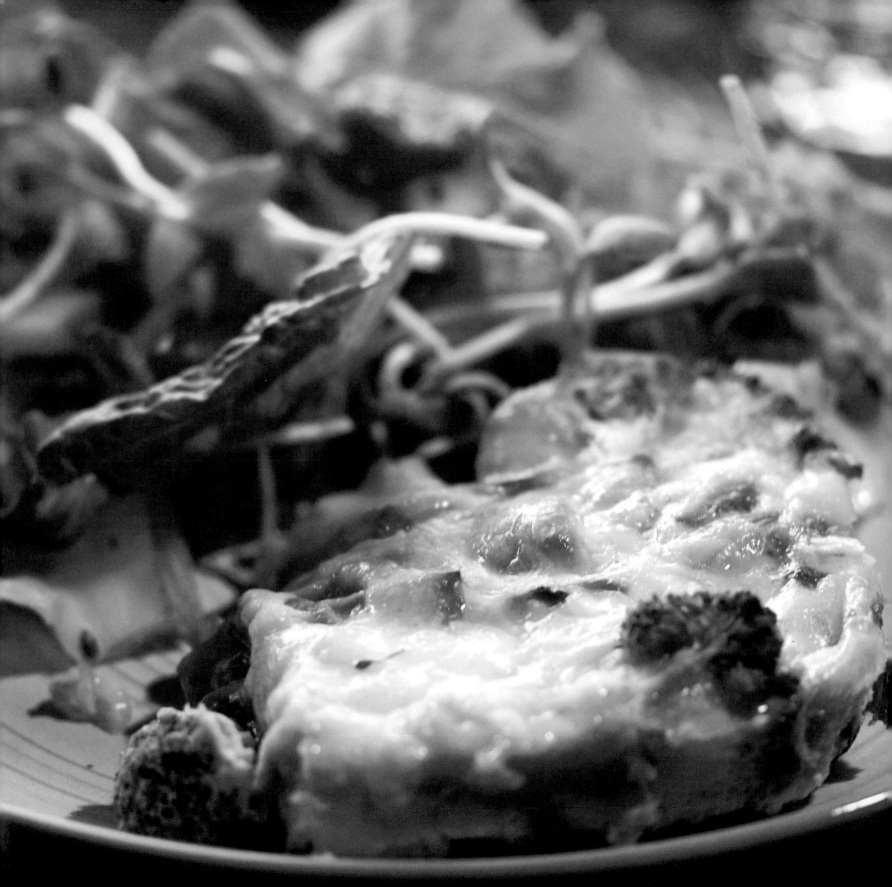

Baby Spinach and Feta Frittata

Ingredients:

1 Tbsp ghee of Gabriel Method-friendly cooking oil
(see page 24)
1 onion, sliced
1 clove garlic, crushed
1 handful of baby spinach leaves
70g feta cheese, cubed (goat's feta is preferable)
2 Tbsp pine nuts
8 eggs (organic, free range), beaten
pinch of healthy salt (see page 17)
¼ cup tasty cheese, grated

Method:

1. Preheat oven to 180°C / 355°F. Grease 20cm square baking dish, lining the base with baking paper.
2. Heat cooking oil in frying pan over medium-high heat.
3. Add onion and cook until it begins to colour. Reduce heat to medium. Add garlic to pan and cook for a further 1-2 minutes. You don't want the garlic to colour or burn.
4. Beat the 8 eggs and salt together in medium bowl.
5. Place baby spinach, feta, pine nuts, onions and garlic in bake tin. Distribute well in the tin then pour egg mix over the top. Sprinkle the grated cheese on top. Cook in oven for 35 minutes or until cooked through.

Smoked Salmon & Courgette Frittata

Ingredients:

1 Tbsp ghee of Gabriel friendly cooking oil
(see page 24)
1 onion, chopped
½ medium zucchini, sliced and quartered
1 clove garlic, crushed
50g smoked salmon, sliced in thin strips
8 eggs (organic, free range), beaten
pinch of healthy salt (see page 17)
¼ cup tasty cheese, grated
1 Tbsp sesame seeds

Method:

1. Preheat oven to 180°C / 355°F. Grease 20cm square baking dish, lining the base with baking paper.
2. Heat cooking oil in frying pan over medium-high heat.
3. Add onion and cook until it begins to colour. Reduce heat to medium. Add zucchini and garlic to pan and cook for a further few minutes. You don't want the garlic to colour or burn.
4. Beat the 8 eggs together with salt in medium bowl.
5. Transfer contents from frying pan to bake tin. Distribute well in the tin. Place smoked salmon strips over mixture then pour egg mix over the top. Cover with the grated cheese and sprinkle with sesame seeds.
6. Cook in oven for 35 minutes or until cooked through.

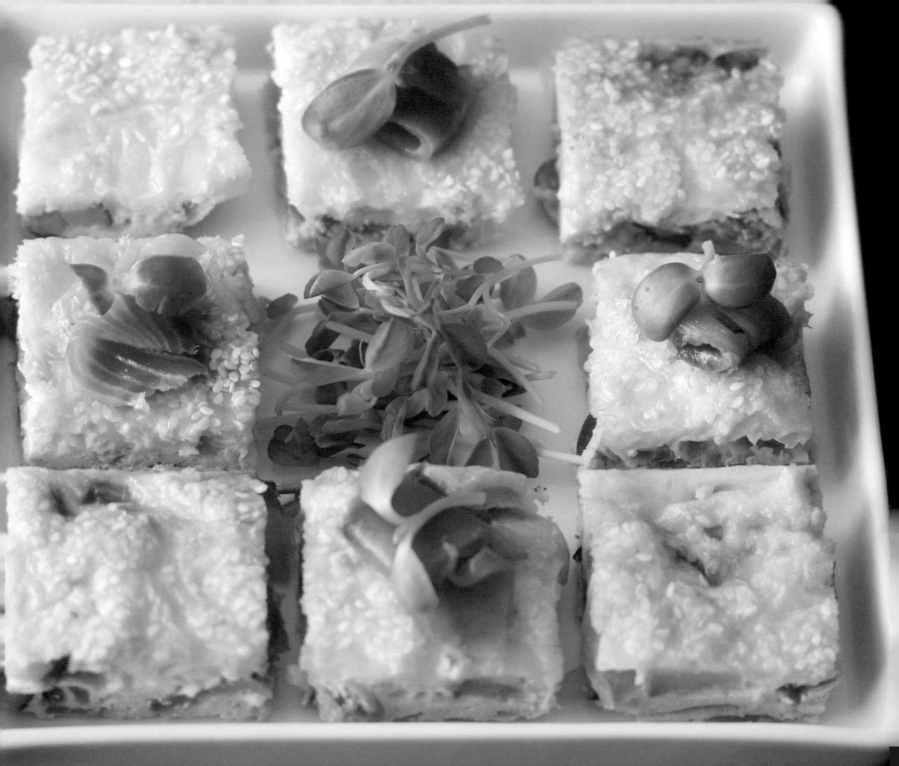

"Shakes and Smoothies are a great way to get the top 3 – Protein, Omega-3s and Live Foods, into a quick, easy and tasty snack that will be loved by kids and adults alike."

Choc Banana Shake

Serves: 1
Preparation time: 5 minutes

Ingredients:
1 banana (frozen if you prefer extra thickness)
1 Tbsp organic cocoa powder
1 egg yolk or 1 Tbsp protein powder
1 Tbsp ground flax seeds
1 tsp xylitol (optional for extra sweetness)
100ml milk, preferably Gabriel Method Nut Milk (see page 256)
contents of 1 probiotic and 1 digestive enzyme capsule (optional)

Method:
Place all ingredients in mixing jug. Mix with stick blender until well combined.

Serve immediately.

Blueberry Smoothie

Serves: 1
Preparation time: 5 minutes

Ingredients:
¾ cup blueberries (frozen for extra thickness)
1 banana, chopped
¾ cup Nut Milk (see page 256) or plain organic yoghurt
1 egg yolk or 1 Tbsp protein powder
1 Tbsp flax seeds, ground
contents of 1 probiotic and 1 digestive enzyme capsule (optional)

Method:
Place all ingredients into a mixing jug. Blend together with stick blender until well combined.

"For a variation, replace the blueberries with your fruit of choice. Some of our favourites include strawberries, mango, raspberries or any combination of these. Make it your own."

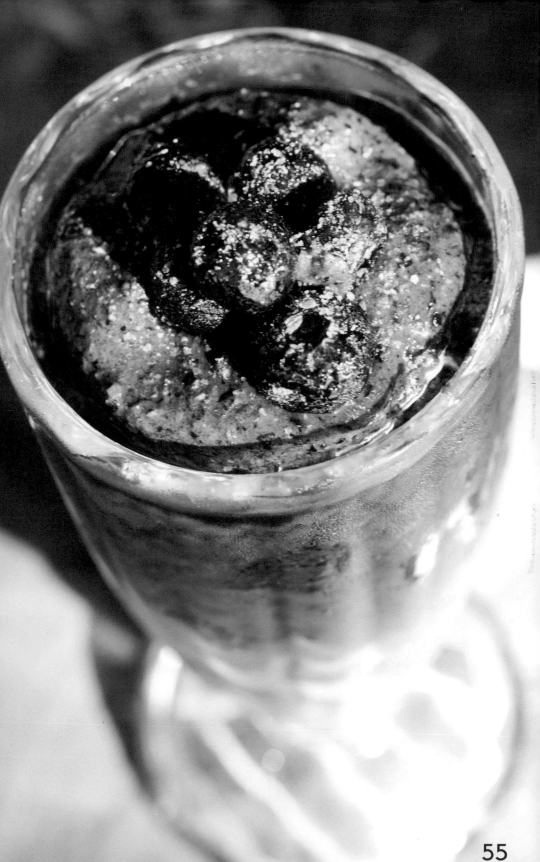

Banana Smoothie

Serves: 1
Preparation time: 5 minutes

Ingredients:
1 banana, chopped (frozen, if you prefer, for added thickness)
1 Tbsp flax seeds, ground
¾ cup plain organic yoghurt
1 egg yolk OR 1 Tbsp protein powder (unflavoured and unsweetened)
contents of 1 probiotic and 1 digestive enzyme capsule (optional)

Method:
Place all ingredients in a mixer jug. Blend with stick blender until well combined.

Spirulina Breaky Smoothie

Serves: 1
Preparation time: 5 minutes

Ingredients:
1 banana, frozen for an extra
thick smoothie
½ cup blueberries, frozen
1 egg yolk or 1 Tbsp protein powder
1 Tbsp spirulina
1 Tbsp flax seeds, ground
10 almonds
¾ cup yoghurt or Gabriel Method nut
milk (see page 256)
contents of 1 probiotic and 1 digestive
enzyme capsule (optional)

Method:
Place all ingredients into a mixing jug.
Blend together with stick blender
until well combined.

*"A funny colour maybe, but
spirulina is full of trace minerals and
nutrients that are very easy for your
body to digest and assimilate. Jon loves
this stuff and is often spotted
sporting his spirulina smile.
Others find the taste rather
challenging, though by mixing it in
with delicious berries, spirulina's
particular flavour can easily be
transformed into a tasty smoothie that
will have you coming back for more."*
– Oona

Snacks and Appetisers

It's natural to snack. It's natural to graze. Three meals a day at set times isn't really how most people have been eating throughout most of human history.

Snacks are really just small meals that your body naturally craves because for most of the time that humans have been on the planet, we've eaten whenever food has been available. Of course, for most of this time virtually endless supplies of food, even poor quality food, hasn't been available. But in the modern world most of us reading this book have access to food readily and easily so there's no real reason to be bound to the arbitrary rule of 'three meals a day'.

Snacking isn't the enemy, but poor choices in snack foods – choices that lead to sugar spikes and sugar crashes – are.

We've included a selection of snacks here, both savoury and sweet, that will keep your blood sugar stable and so kill any cravings in the most satisfying way possible.

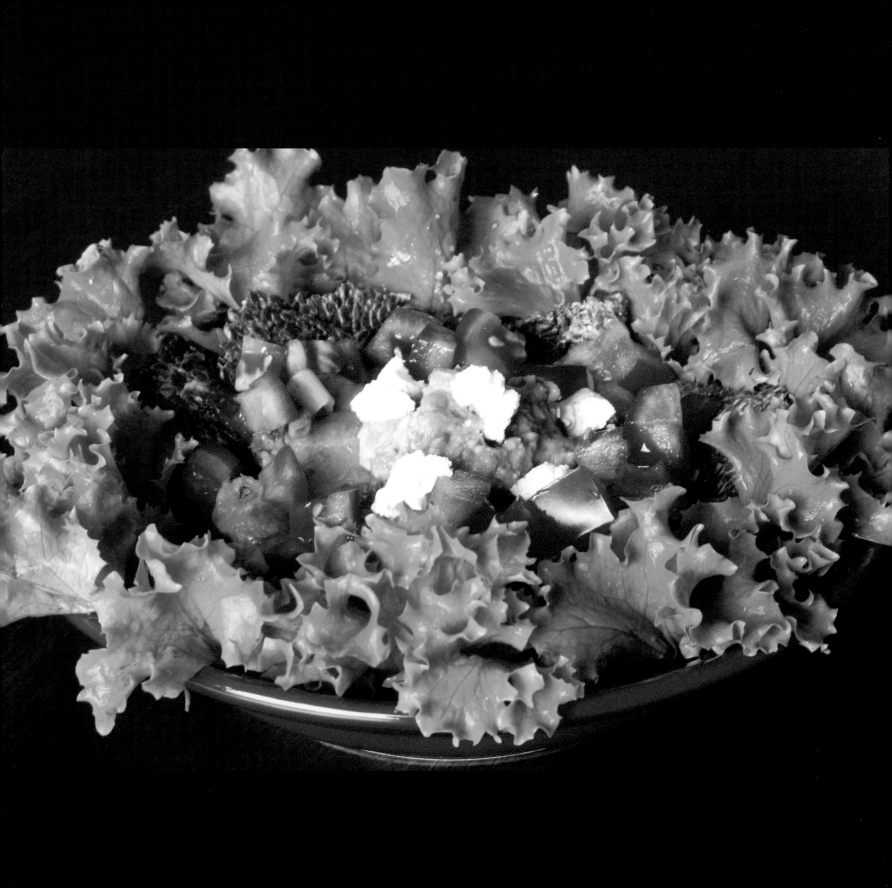

Snacks and Appetisers

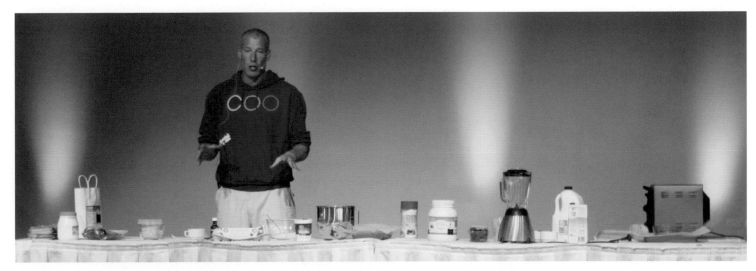

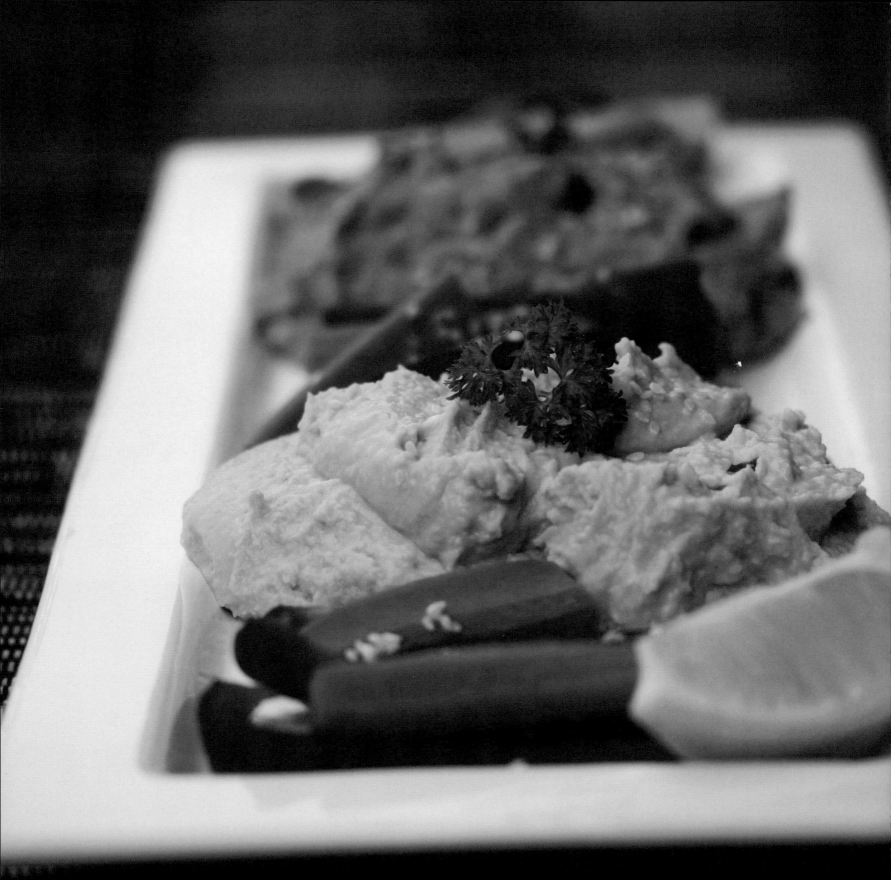

Baba Ganoush

Serves: 6
Preparation time: 10 minutes
Cooking time: 60 minutes

Ingredients:

1 large eggplant
olive oil
healthy salt (see page 17)
2 Tbsp lemon juice

1 clove garlic, crushed
1 Tbsp tahini
1 Tbsp flax seeds
parsley to serve

Method:

1. Cut eggplant in half lengthwise. Place skin side down on baking tray. Paste with olive oil, sprinkle with healthy salt and bake on medium-high heat for 30 minutes or until flesh is cooked.
2. Scoop flesh out of each eggplant segment and put in large bowl.
3. Add lemon juice, crushed garlic, tahini and flax seeds.
4. Blend with stick blender until all combined.
5. Decorate with a parsley sprigs to serve. Serve as a dip with sliced raw veges such as carrot sticks, broccoli pieces or celery sticks or as an accompaniment to lamb dishes.

Hummus

Serves: 6
Preparation time: 5 minutes

Ingredients:

400g chick peas
1 Tbsp tahini
2 Tbsp olive oil
4 Tbsp lemon juice

1 clove garlic
1/4 tsp cumin, ground
1/4 tsp paprika, to serve

Method:

Place all ingredients in a bowl and process with an stick blender until you have a well-combined, smooth consistency. Sprinkle with paprika to serve.

Guacamole

Serves: 6
Preparation time: 10 minutes

Ingredients:
2 avocados
2 cloves garlic
juice of half a lemon
1 tomato, diced
1 Tbsp flax seeds, ground
healthy salt (see page 17) to taste
parsley to serve

Method:
1. Place avocado in a bowl. Mash with a fork to achieve a smooth consistency.
2. Add garlic, lemon juice, diced tomato, flax seeds and salt. Combine ingredients together.
3. Serve with vegetable dipping sticks such as carrot, celery, cucumber.

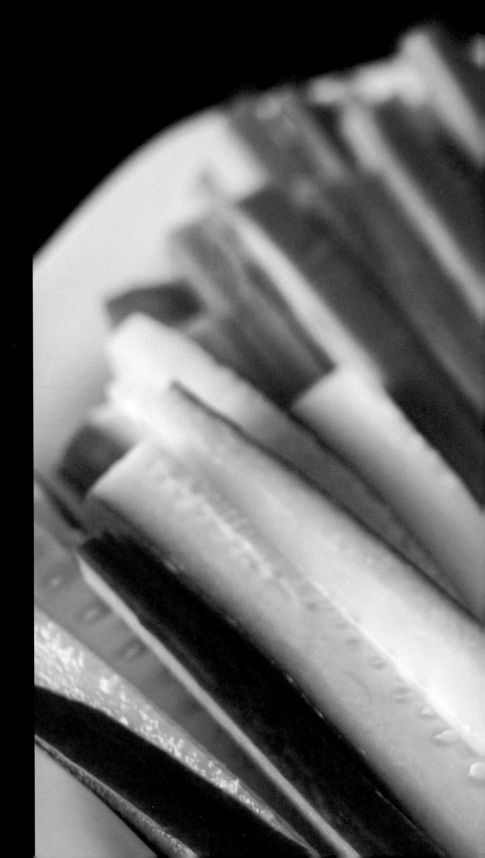

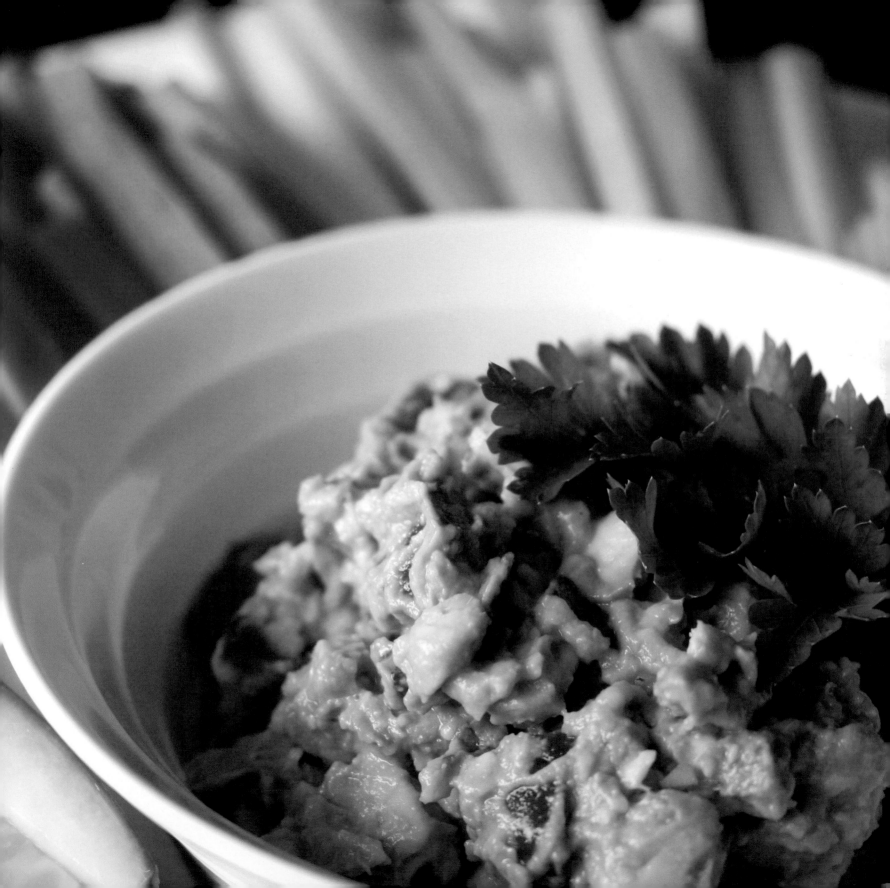

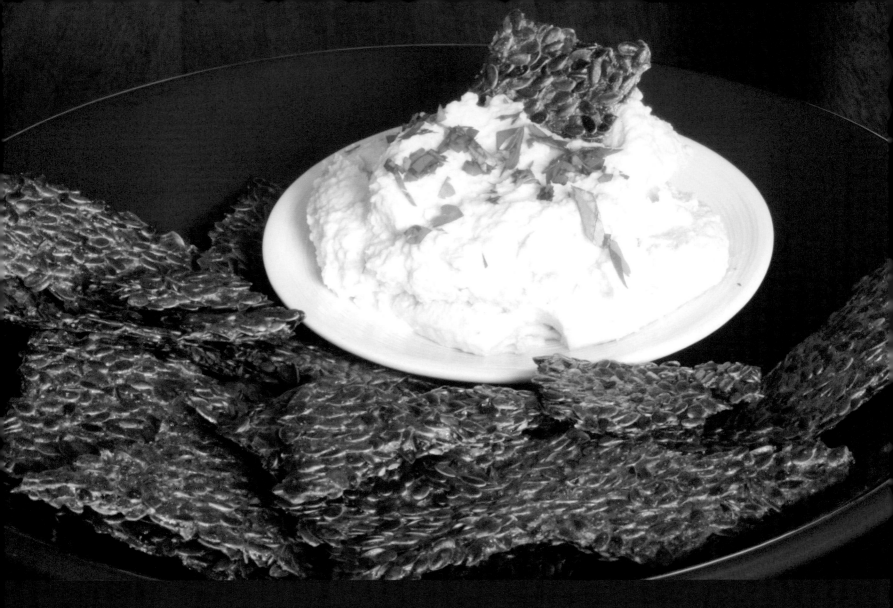

Flax Crackers

Preparation time: 10 minutes
Dehydrating time: Forever! (16 hours :-))

Ingredients:

1 cup flax seeds	1 tsp pepper
1 cup water	1 Tbsp coconut palm sugar
1/2 tsp healthy salt	2 Tbsp olive oil

These Flax Crackers make for great Nachos: just add salsa and your favourite veges then melt cheese over the top and you're good to go. Serve with salad and Gabriel Method Guacomole (see page 64).

Method:
1. Put all ingredients except oil in a bowl.
2. Blend for a few minutes with a stick blender until gelatinous.
3. Spread onto dehydrator sheet.
4. Add oil on top to help with spreading.
5. Spread as thin and uniform as possible without any gaps.
6. Dehydrate 1 hour. Take out and score into squares or triangles.
7. Dehydrate for another 12-14 hours at 40°C / 105°F.
8. Flip and dehydrate for 2-4 more hours until crunchy.

Cauli Mash

Serves: 4
Preparation time: 10 minutes
Cooking time: 10 minutes

Ingredients:
1 cauliflower, cut into florets
pinch nutmeg
1 Tbsp butter
salt and pepper to taste

Method:
To prepare the cauliflower, place cauliflower florets in a medium saucepan with water. Boil until cauliflower softens. Transfer cauliflower to medium mixing bowl. Add butter and blend with hand held blender until mashed. Add nutmeg and season with salt, gently stir in. Cover to keep warm.

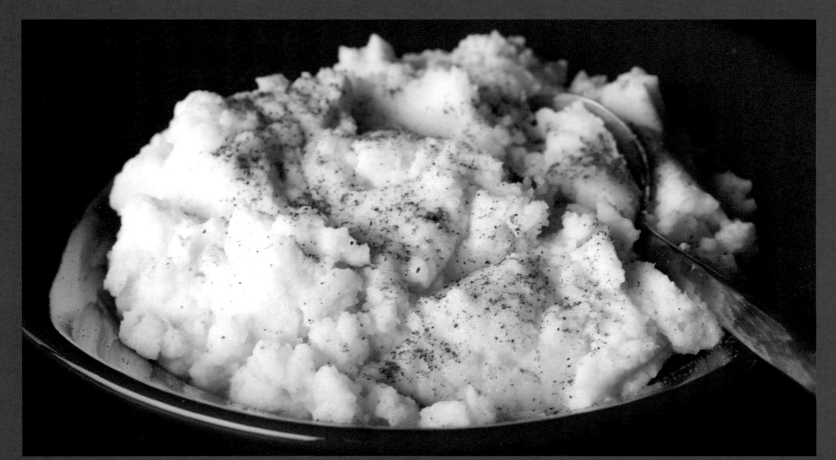

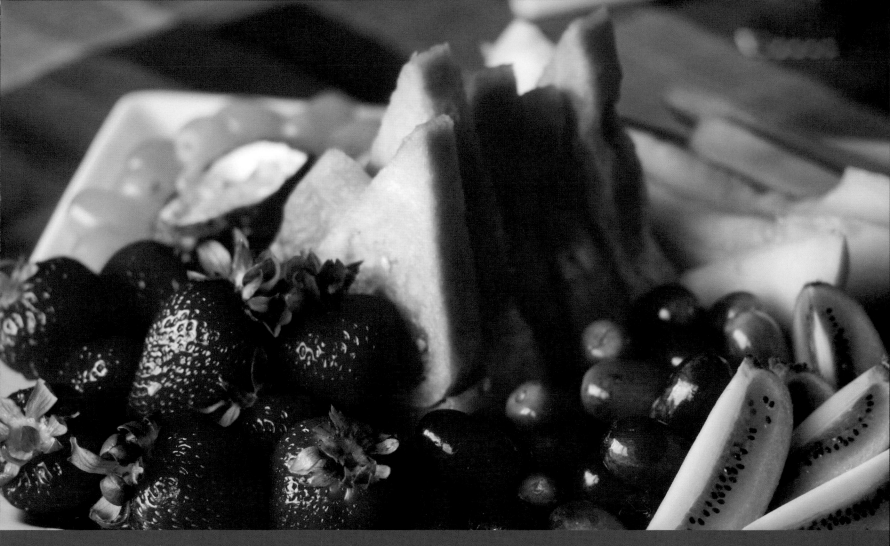

Fruit Platter

Serves: 6
Preparation time: 15 minutes

Ingredients:

¼ of a watermelon, cut into wedges

¼ of a honeydew melon, cut into wedges

2 kiwi fruit, quartered lengthways

2 passionfruits, halved

1 mango, cut into thin strips

12 strawberries

1 medium bunch green grapes

1 medium bunch red grapes

Method:

1. Wash all fruit prior to cutting
2. Arrange cut fruit onto a platter.

Corn Thin Faces

Makes: 12
Preparation time: 10 minutes

Ingredients:
12 organic corn thin crackers
1 avocado
6 Tbsp hummus
½ cucumber, thinly sliced and halved
½ red capsicum (bell pepper), thinly sliced lengthways
12 cherry tomatoes, halved
cheddar cheese, cut into small triangles
sprouts or broccoli for the hair

Method:
1. Give each corn thin a base layer of either hummus or avocado.
2. Using the different vegetables, create various funny faces. Or give them to the kids to decorate. They'll love the creative process and will be even more enthusiastic to eat them up.

"Get the kids involved with this one. They'll love putting different facial expressions on their corn thins using the fresh and colourful toppings."

Please note: This is the only recipe in the book that contains gluten.

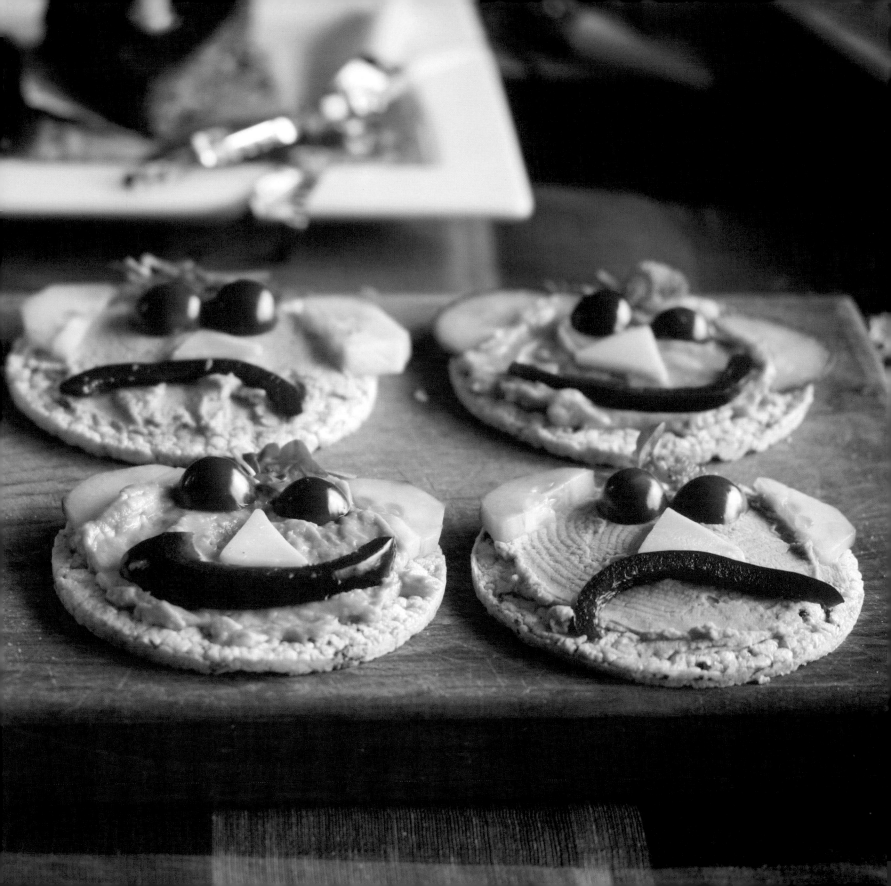

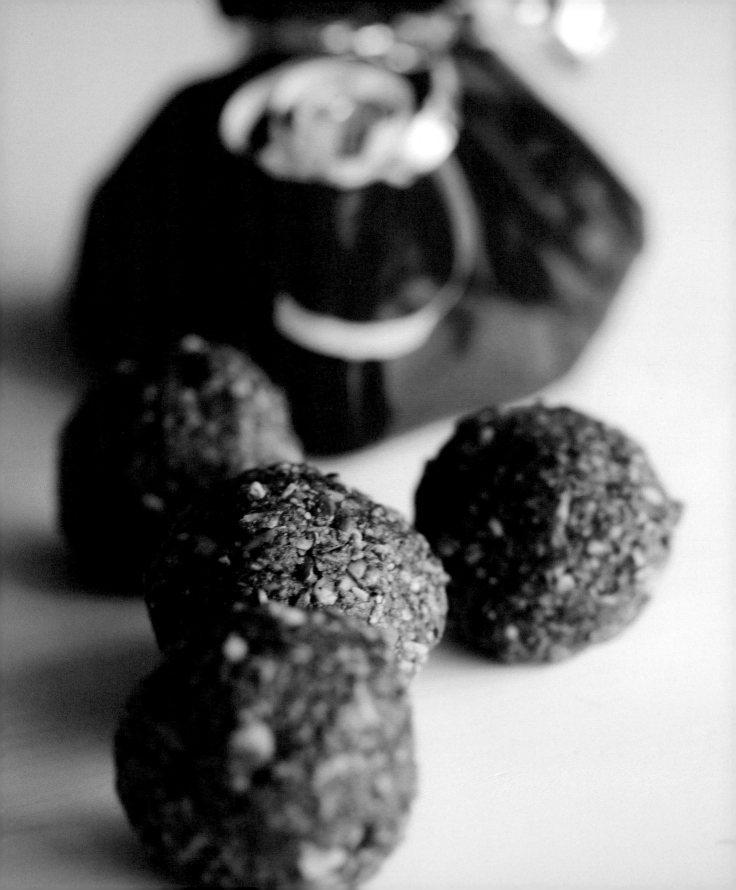

Choc Seed Treats

Makes: 10
Preparation time: 15 minutes

Ingredients:
⅓ cup almonds
1 Tbsp sunflower seeds
1 Tbsp pumpkin seeds
1 Tbsp organic desiccated coconut
1 Tbsp flax seeds
1 tsp sesame seeds
1 Tbsp cocoa powder
1 tsp cinnamon
3 Tbsp almond butter
1 Tbsp tahini
1½ tsp coconut palm sugar
1½ tsp xylitol

A special treat, great for after school snacks, blood sugar leveliser, or wrap in pretty paper and offer as a gift.

Method:
1. Place all ingredients in a food processor. Mix until mixture begins to stick together.
2. Roll mixture into small balls, approximately 1 Tbsp of mixture per ball.
3. Eat instantly or refrigerate until you feel ready for this scrumptious treat.

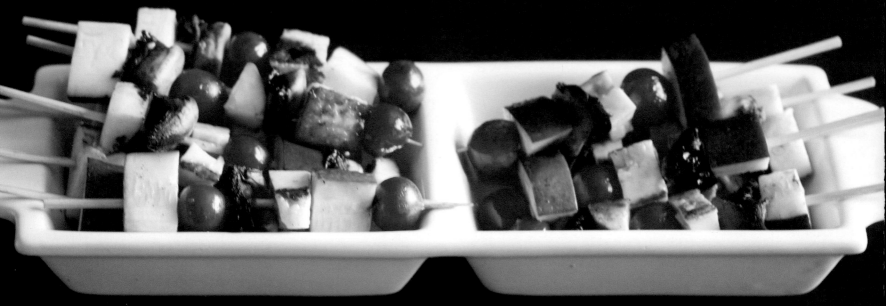

Grilled Haloumi Kebabs

Makes: 15
Preparation time: 20 minutes
Cooking time: 5 minutes

Ingredients:
15 small kebab sticks (soak in water prior to using)
100g haloumi, cubed
½ zucchini, cut into bite size pieces
30 cherry tomatoes
4 mushrooms, quartered
Gabriel friendly cooking oil (see page 24)

Method:
1. Thread food pieces onto kebab sticks.
2. Heat cooking oil on grill or BBQ. Cook kebabs, turning them so that each side gets cooked.
3. Remove from heat and serve instantly. So delicious!

Party Meatballs

Makes: Approximately 20 meatballs
Preparation time: 20 minutes
Cooking time: 10 minutes

Ingredients:
500g organic grass fed beef, minced (ground)
1 egg yolk
1 small onion, finely diced
1 Tbsp thyme leaves, fresh or dried
healthy salt (see page 17) and pepper
to season
2 Tbsp Gabriel friendly cooking oil
(see page 24)

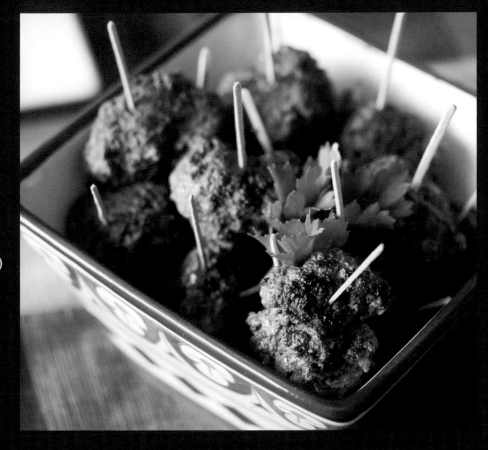

Method:
1. To make the meatballs, place all ingredients in a bowl and mix with hands or wooden spoon to combine. With wet hands, shape the meat mixture into balls. The mixture should make approximately 20 meatballs.
2. Heat 1 Tbsp cooking oil in a frying pan on medium to high heat. Place half the meatballs into the pan and cook, turning until browned all over and cooked through. Repeat with remaining oil and meatballs.
3. Transfer to a serving plate and insert a toothpick into each meatballs.
4. Serve with Gabriel Method Tomato Sauce or Gabriel Method Chilli Tahini Sauce (see pages 200 and 206).

Prawn Parcels

Serves: 4
Preparation time: 20 minutes
Cooking time: 5 minutes for prawns (shrimp)

Ingredients:
1 red capsicum (bell pepper), seeded, cut into small cubes
1 cucumber, cut into small cubes
2 spring onions (scallions) (scallions) sliced
2 tsp lime juice
2 tsp tamari
1½ Tbsp hoisin sauce
8 baby cos lettuce (romaine) leaves
750g prawns (shrimp), cooked and peeled
1 Tbsp flax seeds

Method:
1. In a medium bowl combine capsicum (bell pepper), cucumber, spring onions (scallions), lime juice, tamari and hoisin sauce. Stir together well.
2. Place the lettuce leaves onto serving plates. Evenly distribute the capsicum and cucumber mixture amongst the lettuce leaves. Top each parcel with cooked prawns (shrimp). Sprinkle with ground flax seeds and serve.

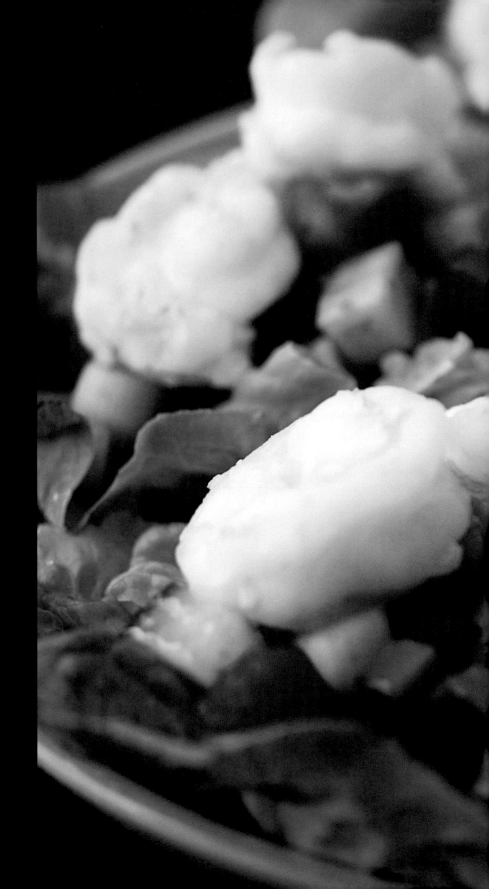

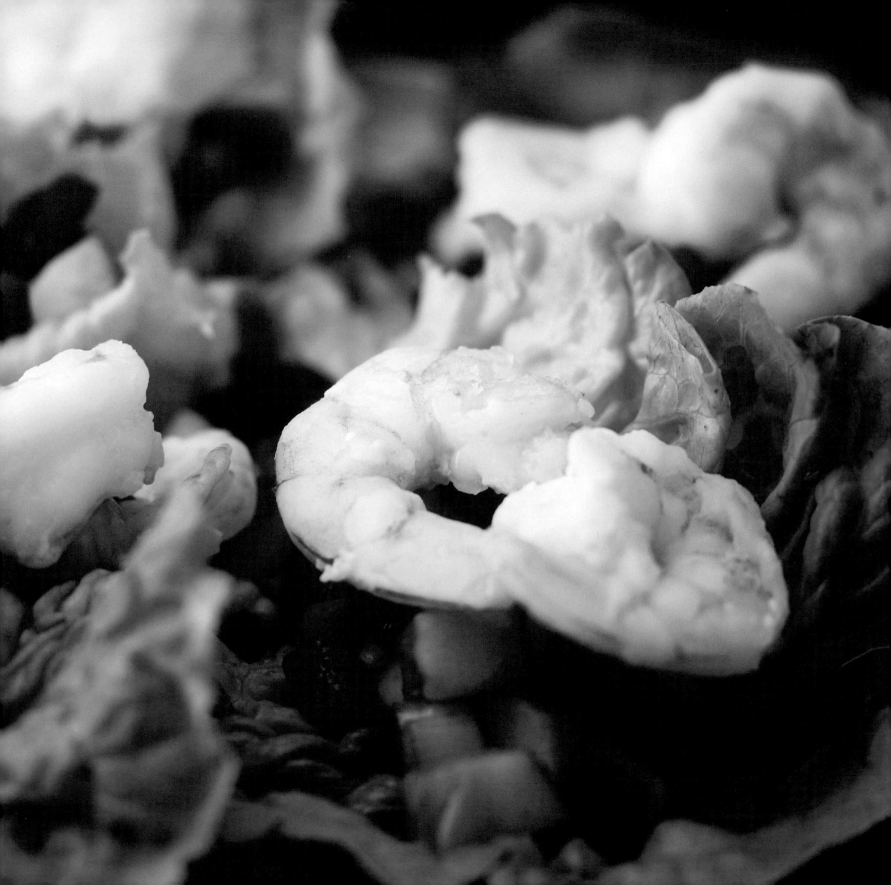

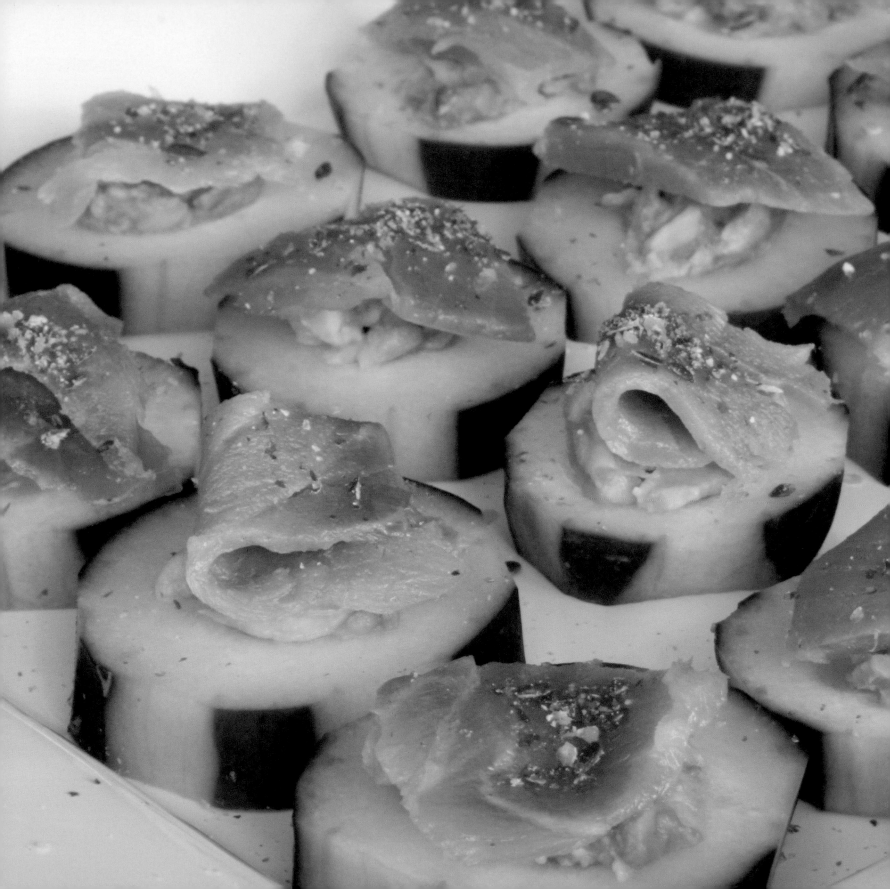

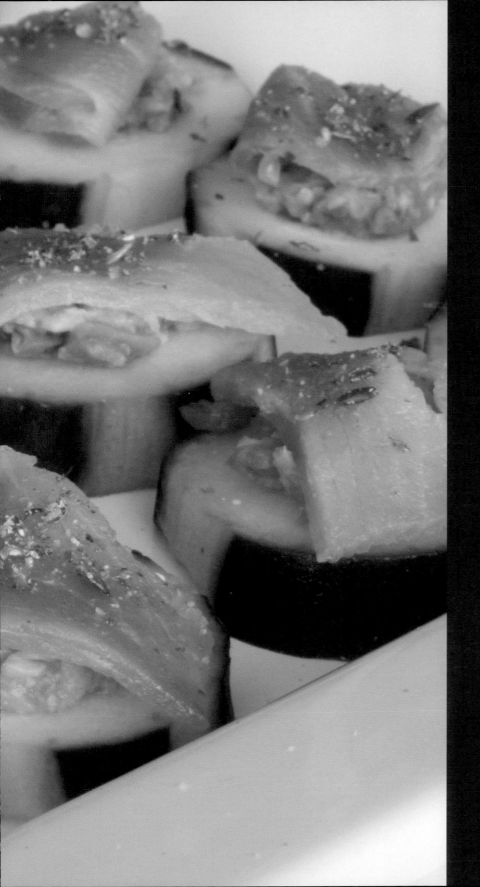

Cucumber Bites

Makes: 25-25
Preparation time: 15 minutes

Ingredients:
1 Lebanese cucumber, cut into 1cm rounds
1 avocado
150g smoked salmon
2 tsp ground flax seeds

Method:
1. Place cucumber slices on large serving plate.
2. Top each cucumber slice with a small dab of avocado topped with a slice of smoked salmon.
3. Sprinkle with flax seeds and serve.

"A light and tasty finger food. Cucumber makes for a clever cracker convert."

Smoked Turkey Cranberry Bites

Makes: 20
Preparation time: 15 minutes

Ingredients:
225g smoked turkey (or chicken), sliced into 20 x 5mm slices
2 small avocados, sliced lengthways
40g (50mls) cranberry sauce*

*If making your own cranberry sauce, try to replace the sugar with Gabriel Method-friendly sweeteners (see page 25).

Method:
Place smoked turkey slices on a serving plate. Top each piece of turkey with a slice of avocado and ½ tsp of cranberry sauce. Serve with drinks at Thanksgiving or Christmas celebrations.

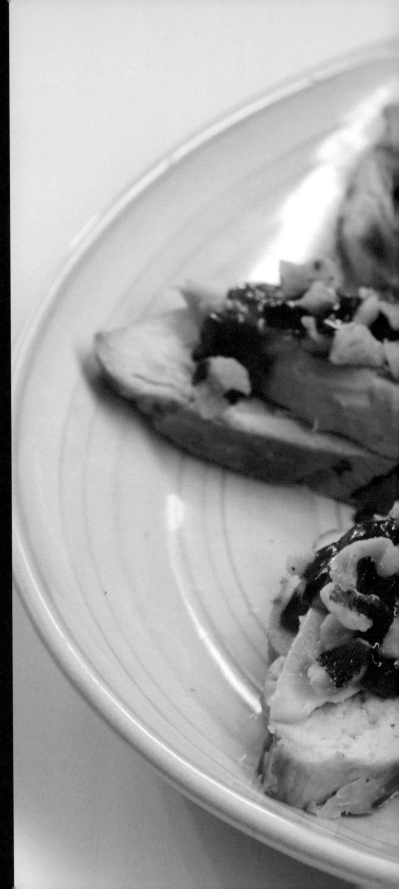

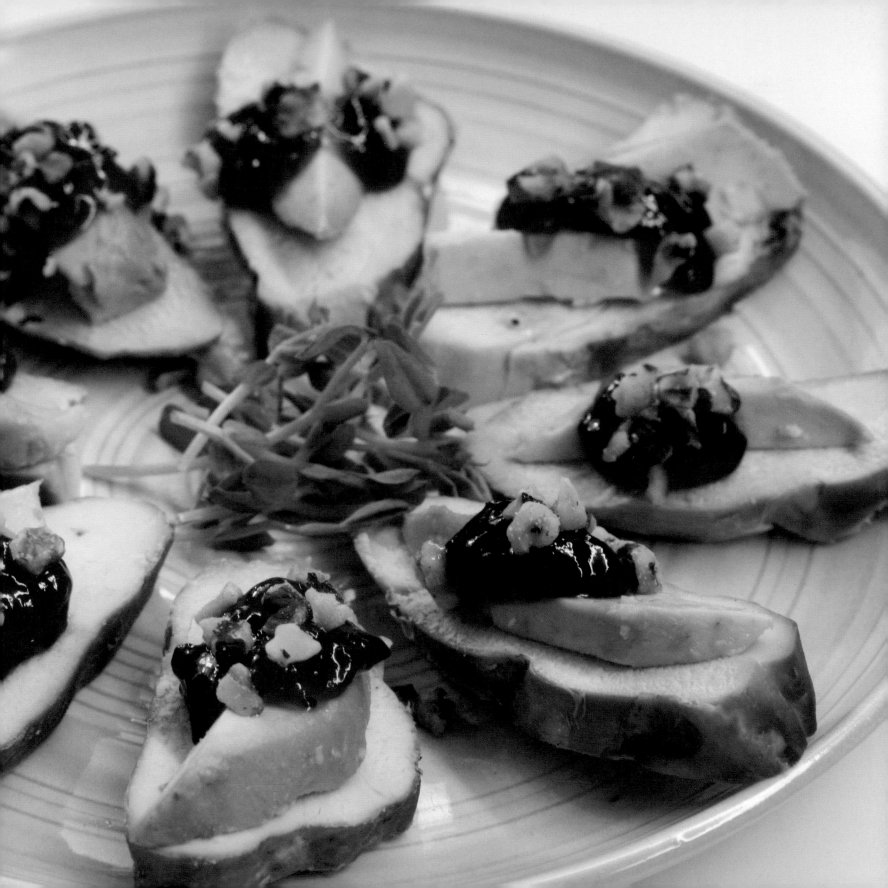

Muesli Balls

Makes: 35
Preparation Time: 30 minutes

Ingredients:
1½ cups almonds
⅓ cup pumpkin seeds
¾ cup sunflower seeds
¼ cup sesame seeds
¾ cup desiccated coconut
1 cup flax seeds
½ cup almond butter
⅓ cup water
⅓ cup tahini
¼ cup coconut palm sugar
¼ cup xylitol

Method:
1. Place all ingredients in food processor. Mix together until well combined and beginning to stick together.
2. Roll mixture into small balls, approximately 2 tablespoons of mixture per ball.
3. Eat instantly or refrigerate in an airtight container.

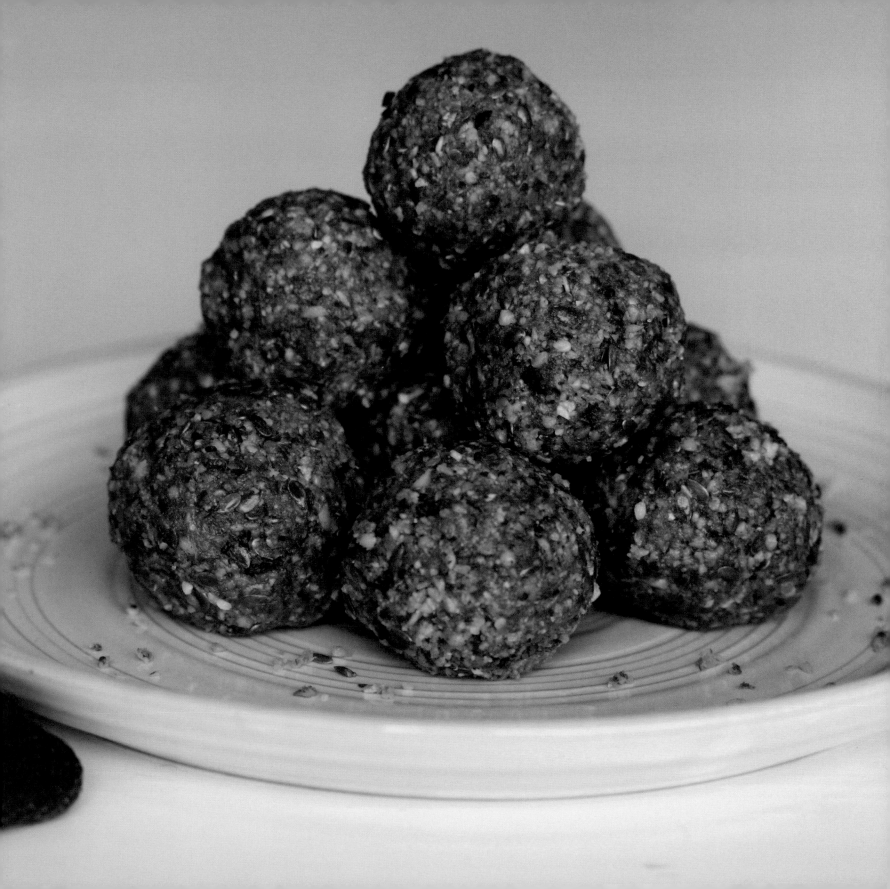

Cauli Nori Rolls

Makes: 6 rolls
Preparation time: 30 minutes

Ingredients:
6 nori sheets
½ cauliflower
½ cup almonds
1 tsp tamari
juice of ½ a lemon

Fillings:

avocado	egg
cucumber	prawns (shrimp)
sprouts	crab
smoked salmon	pickled ginger
chicken	wasabi
tuna	

Method:
1. In a food processor, mix together cauliflower, almonds, tamari and lemon juice. Process until well combined.
2. Lay out nori sheet with shiny side face down. Place ¼ cup of cauliflower mix onto nori sheet. Spread it out thinly, reaching to both sides of sheet and about 7 cm along the sheet. Place chosen toppings in a strip in middle of cauliflower, reaching to both sides of sheet.
3. Roll the nori sheet over the toppings until the entire sheet is rolled up. With dampened fingers, moisten the edge of nori sheet to assist with sticking it to itself. Cut roll into 6 even pieces.
4. Repeat with remaining nori sheets and toppings.

This is a great way to make super delicious sushi rolls without the rice

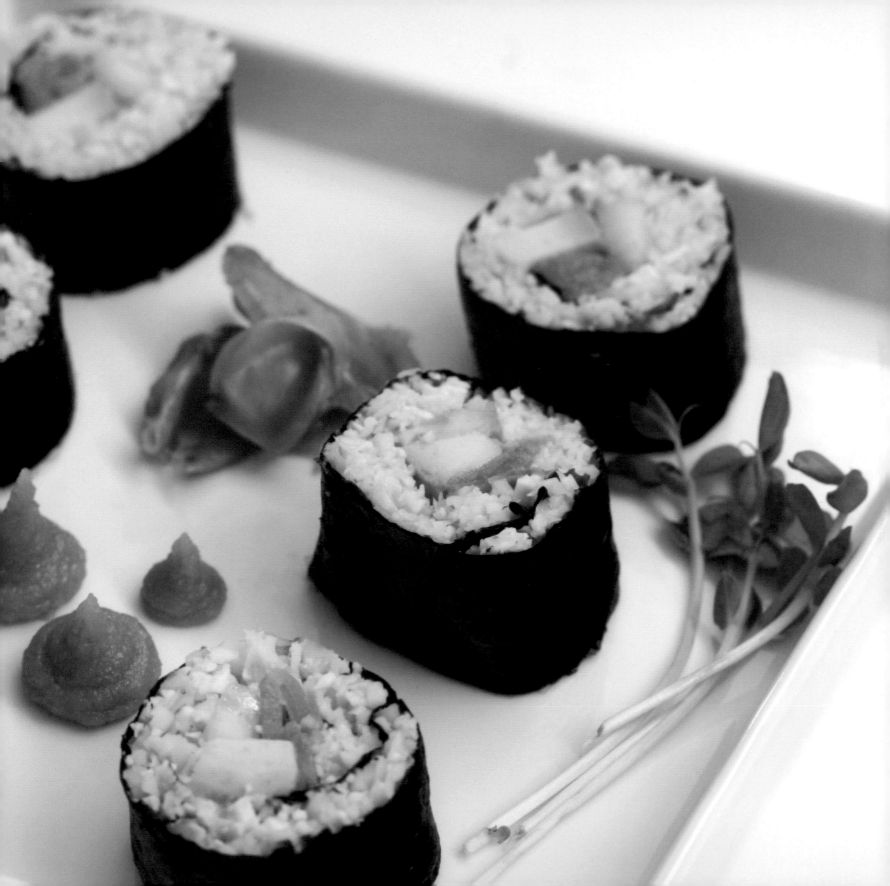

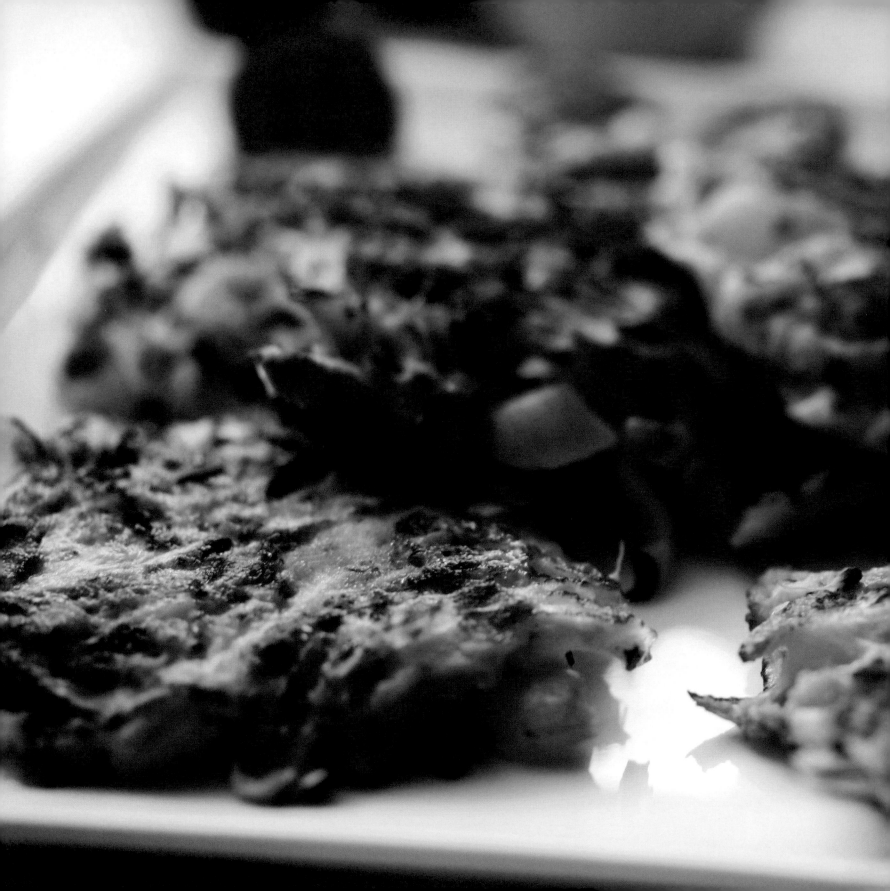

Vege Fritters

Makes: 8
Preparation time: 10 minutes
Cooking time: 15 minutes

Ingredients:
2 Tbsp Gabriel friendly cooking oil (see page 24)
1 small brown onion, diced
30g broccoli, finely chopped
1 clove garlic, crushed
⅓ cup carrot, grated
⅓ cup zucchini, grated
1 egg
1 tsp thyme
salt and pepper

Method:
1. Heat cooking oil in frying pan on medium heat.
2. Place diced onion, broccoli and garlic in frying pan. Cook for approximately 3 minutes. Remove from heat.
3. Beat egg in medium bowl. Transfer onion, broccoli and garlic from frying pan to bowl. Add carrot, zucchini, thyme, salt and pepper. Mix until well combined and everything is coated in egg.
4. Wipe the frying pan clean with kitchen paper. Heat 1 Tbsp cooking oil in frying pan to prevent sticking. Place dessert spoon sized scoops of mixture into frying pan. Scoop from the bottom of the bowl to be sure you are getting egg in your scoop. Cook 2 minutes on each side or until lightly browned. Wipe the frying pan clean and reapply cooking oil between batches.
5. Serve sprinkled with flax seeds.

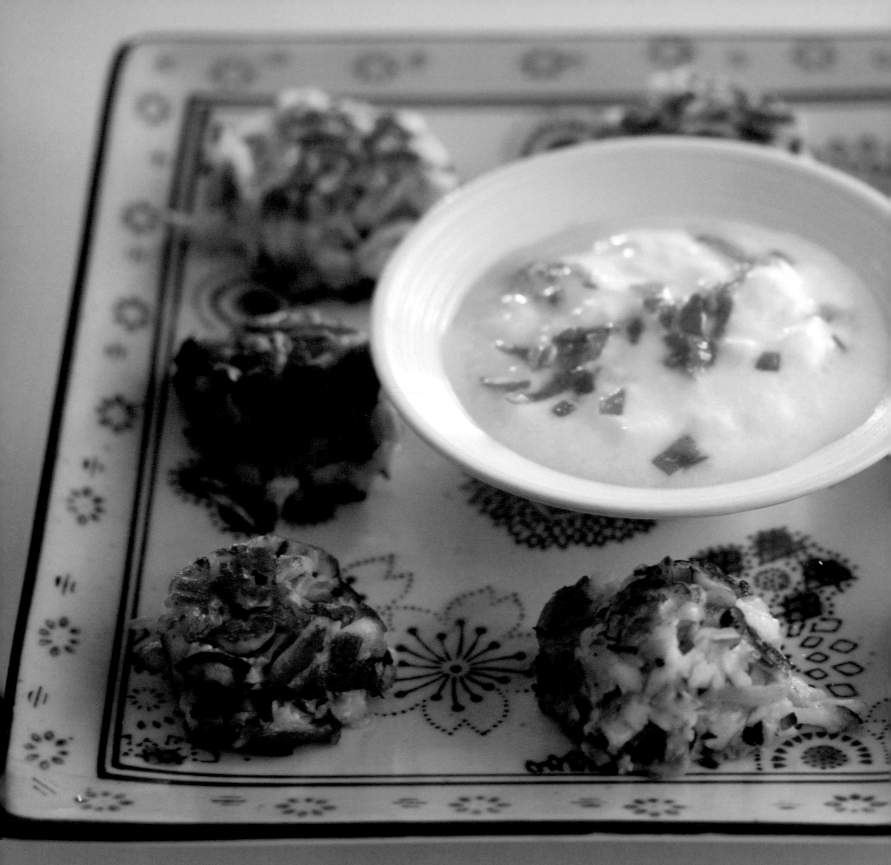

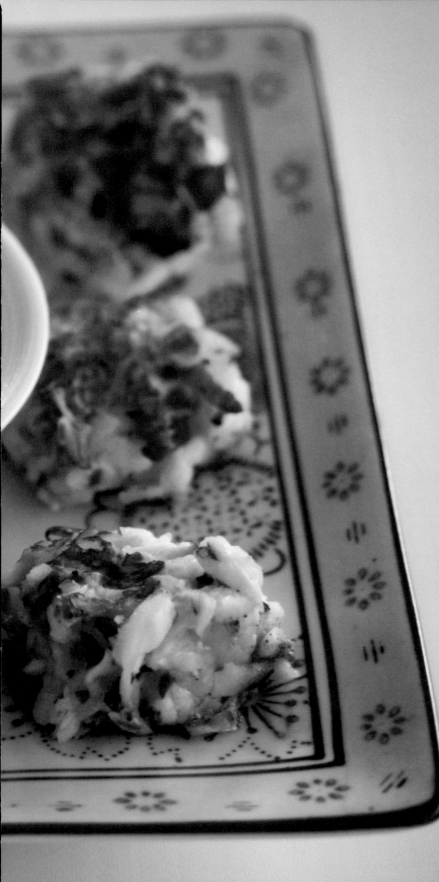

Zucchini & Haloumi Fritters

Makes: 20
Preparation time: 15 minutes
Cooking time: 20 minutes

Ingredients:
2 zucchinis, grated
180g haloumi, grated
2 spring onions (scallions), cut finely
2 eggs (organic, free range), beaten
salt and pepper to season
2 Tbsp Gabriel Method friendly-cooking oil
(see page 24)

Yoghurt Dipping Sauce:
½ cup yoghurt
1 Tbsp lemon juice
1 clove garlic, crushed
1 Tbsp flax seeds, ground
1 Tbsp fresh chives, cut finely

Method:
1. Place grated zucchini into clean tea towel and squeeze it over the sink to reduce liquid content.
2. Combine zucchini with haloumi, spring onions, eggs, salt and pepper. Mix together well.
3. Heat cooking oil in frying pan on medium to high heat. Form the mixture into small balls in the palm of your hand, approximately 1 tablespoon per ball. Squeeze any excess liquid out of them.
4. Cook in batches in frying pan for 2-3 minutes on each side or until golden brown and cooked through. Wipe frying pan clean with absorbant paper between batches and reapply oil.
5. Serve warm with yoghurt dipping sauce.

89

Bite Size Frittatas

Makes: 12

Feta and Chives
Preparation time: 10 minutes
Cooking time: 10 minutes

Ingredients:

2 eggs (organic, free range), beaten
20g feta cheese, diced

1 Tbsp chives, cut finely
¼ cup cheddar cheese, grated (optional)

Method:
1. Preheat oven to 180°C / 355°F.
2. Place beaten eggs, feta and chives into medium bowl with spout. Pour contents into mini muffin tray. Evenly distribute grated cheese on top of each mini omelette.
3. Bake in oven for 10 minutes or until lightly browned on top.

Ham and Onion
Preparation time: 10 minutes
Cooking time: 15 minutes

Ingredients:

2 eggs (organic, free range), beaten
1 slice ham (organic grass-fed), diced
½ small onion, diced

¼ cup cheddar cheese, grated (optional)
1 Tbsp Gabriel friendly cooking oil
(see page 24)

Method:
Preheat oven to 180°C / 355°F.
1. Heat cooking oil in frying pan on medium to high heat. Cook diced onion for 3 minutes or until it is lightly browned.
2. Place beaten eggs, ham and onion into medium bowl with spout. Pour contents into mini muffin tray. Evenly distribute grated cheese on top of each Bite Size Frittata.
3. Bake in oven for 10 minutes or until lightly browned on top.

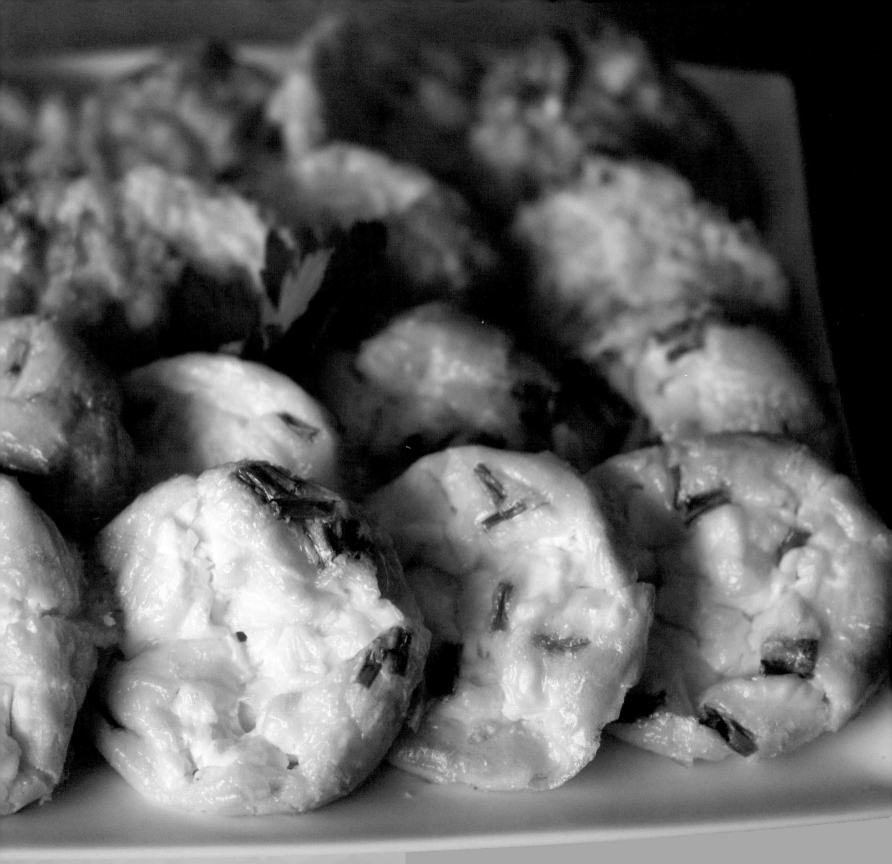

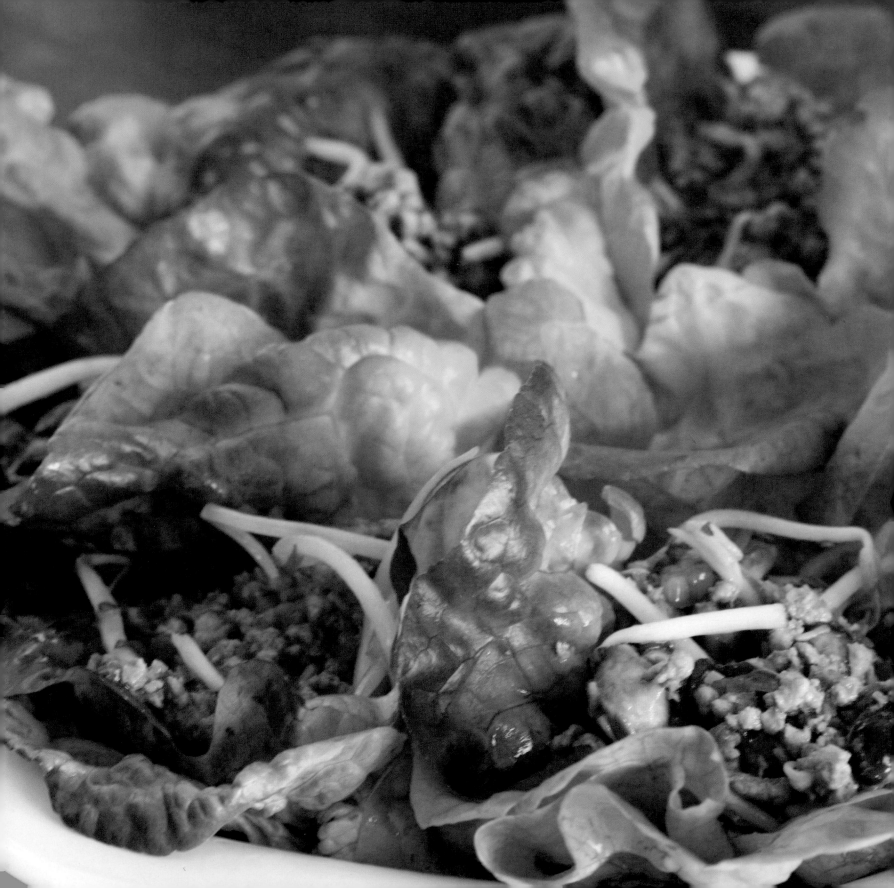

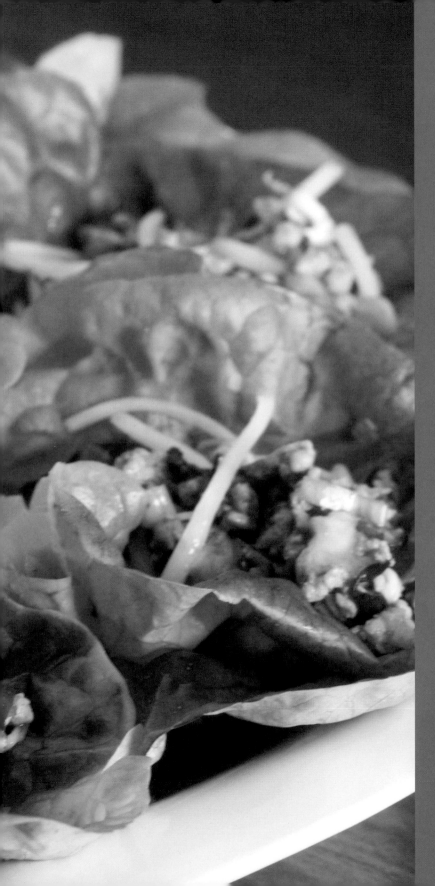

Sang Choy Bow

Serves: 12-15 servings
Preparation time: 15 minutes
Cooking time: 15 minutes

Ingredients:
1 Tbsp sesame oil
500g lean pork mince
1 small brown onion, chopped finely
1 clove garlic, crushed
1cm fresh ginger, grated
2 Tbsp water
100g shiitake mushrooms
2 Tbsp tamari
2 Tbsp oyster sauce
1 Tbsp lime juice
2 cups bean sprouts
4 spring onions (scallions), thinly sliced
¼ cup fresh coriander, coarsely chopped
12 large butter lettuce leaves
2 Tbsp flax seeds, ground

Method:
1. Heat oil in wok or large frying pan on medium heat. Add onion, garlic and ginger. Cook for 1-2 minutes or until beginning to brown. Add pork and stir until it changes colour.
2. Add water, mushrooms, tamari, oyster sauce and lime juice. Stir fry until mushrooms are just tender. Remove from heat. Add sprouts, spring onions (scallions) and coriander. Lightly stir through to combine.
3. Place lettuce leaves on a serving plate. Spoon even amounts of pork mixture onto each lettuce leaf. Sprinkle with flax seeds and serve.

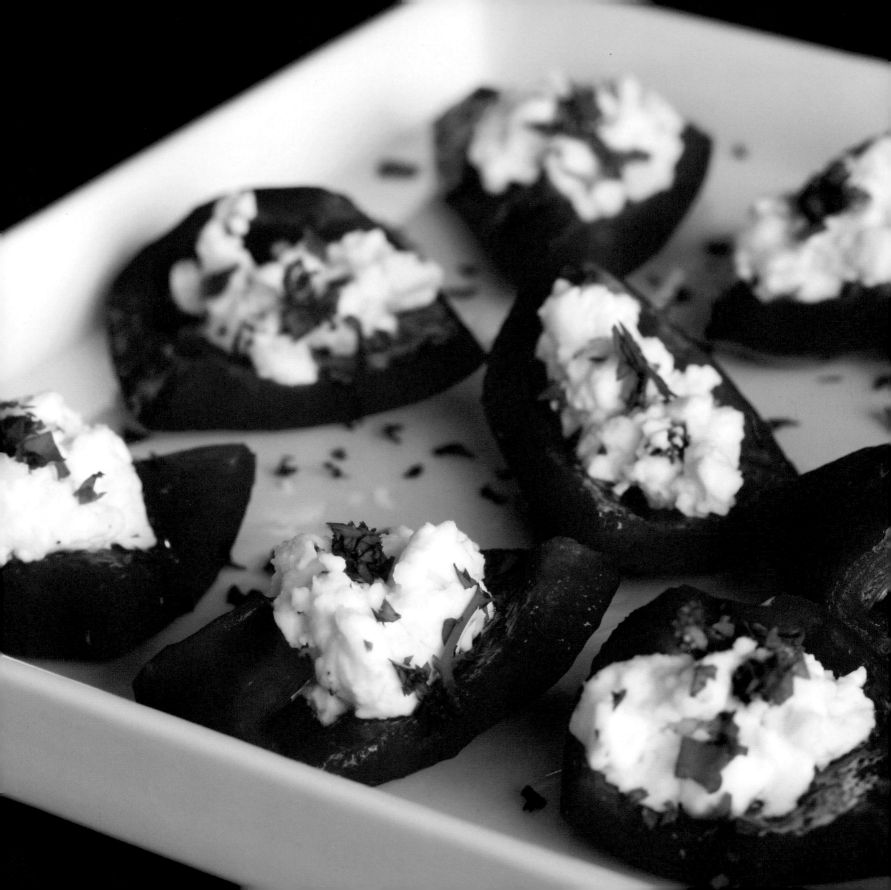

Red Capsicum (bell pepper) and Goat's Cheese Nibbles

Makes: 12 – 16
Preparation time: 15 minutes
Cooking time: 20 minutes

Ingredients:
1 medium red capsicum (bell pepper)
1 tsp Gabriel friendly cooking oil (see page 24)
100g soft goat's cheese
1 tsp thyme leaves
healthy salt (see page 17) and pepper to taste
1 Tbsp parsley, finely chopped

Method:
1. Preheat the oven to 180°C / 355°F.
2. Cut the capsicum (bell pepper) lengthways into
   4 pieces, discarding core and seeds.
   Place capsicum pieces on a baking tray. Drizzle
   with cooking oil and bake in oven for 6-8
   minutes until they become tender.
3. In a mixing bowl, place goat's cheese, thyme,
   salt and pepper. Stir together until
   well combined.
4. Remove capsicum from oven. Cut each piece
   into 3 or 4 bite-size portions. Divide goat's
   cheese mixture between the capsicum pieces.
   Bake in oven for a further 2-3 minutes until
   cheese is warm. Garnish with finely chopped
   parsley prior to serving.

Prawn Cocktail

Serves: 4
Preparation time: 20 minutes if peeling and cleaning prawns (shrimp) yourself
Cooking time: 5 minutes

Ingredients:
1 kg peeled raw wild prawns (shrimp) with tails attached
1 Tbsp Gabriel Method-friendly cooking oil
Nicoise Dressing (page 205)

Method:
1. Heat cooking oil in frying pan on a high heat. Add prawns (shrimp) and cook for 3-5 minutes or until prawns are completely white with pink markings.
2. Serve prawns hot with fresh lettuce and Niçoise Dressing (see page 205).

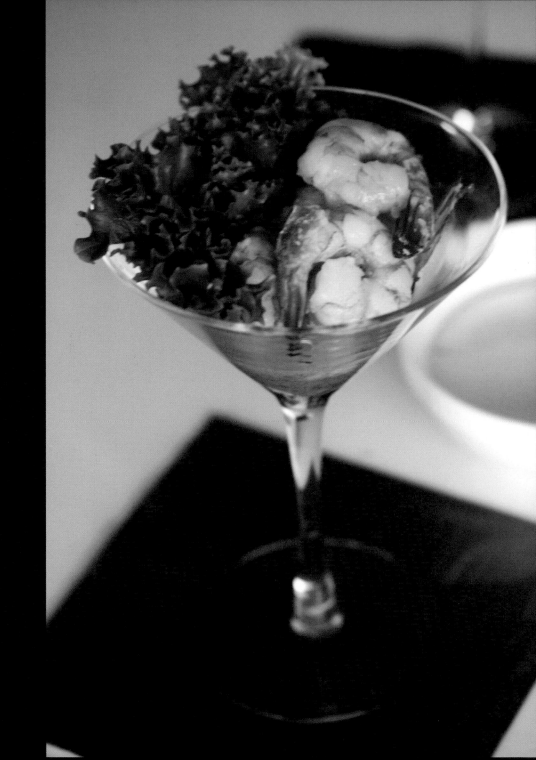

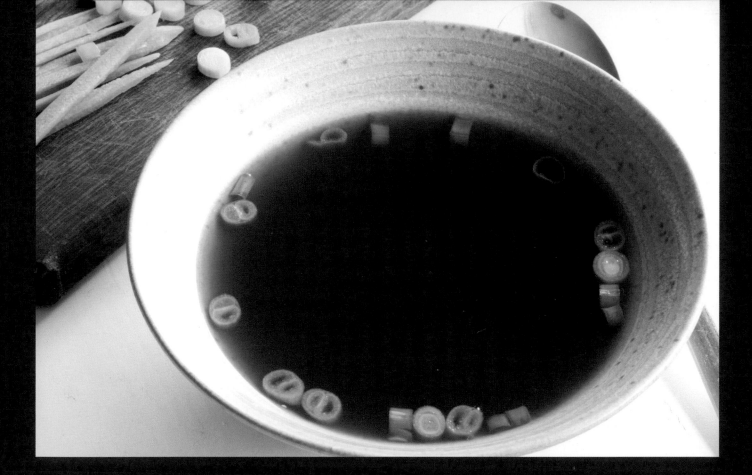

Miso Soup

Serves: 1
Preparation time: 5 minutes
Cooking time: 5 minutes

Ingredients:

1 Tbsp organic miso paste
1 cup of water
chopped spring onions (scallions)

Miso soup makes for a great light meal or satisfying quick snack. Made from soybeans, miso is a natural fermented product with many nutritional benefits. There are many types of miso, so experiment with a few to find your favourite. Miso can also be sold as a powder to be mixed with hot water. If you purchase it in this form, check the packaging to be sure there are no added baddies, such as MSG, artificial colours or preservatives.

Method:

1. Boil water and stir in miso paste, add spring onions (scallions) and serve.

*Add cooked chicken, meat or fish and veges, for a more substantial Miso.

Baked Ricotta

Serves: 4
Preparation time: 10 minutes
Cooking time: 30 minutes

Ingredients:
1 Tbsp ghee or Gabriel friendly oil (see page 24)
500g ricotta
2 eggs (organic, free range)
½ cup chives
1 tsp chilli flakes (optional)
healthy salt (see page 17) and pepper

Method:
1. Preheat oven to 180°C / 355°F.
2. Grease 4 x 125ml ramekins.
3. In a bowl, combine ricotta, eggs, chives, chilli flakes, salt and pepper.
4. Distribute mixture into ramekins smoothing the surface with the back of a spoon.
5. Bake in oven for 30 minutes or until golden brown on surface.
6. Allow to cool a while before serving.

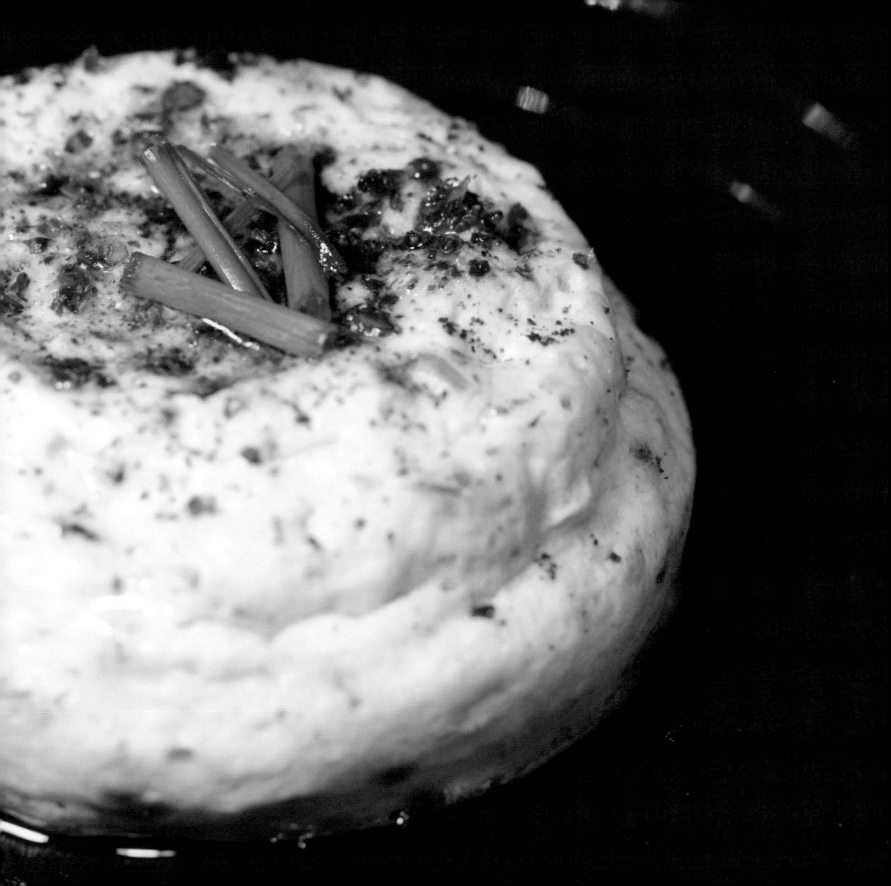

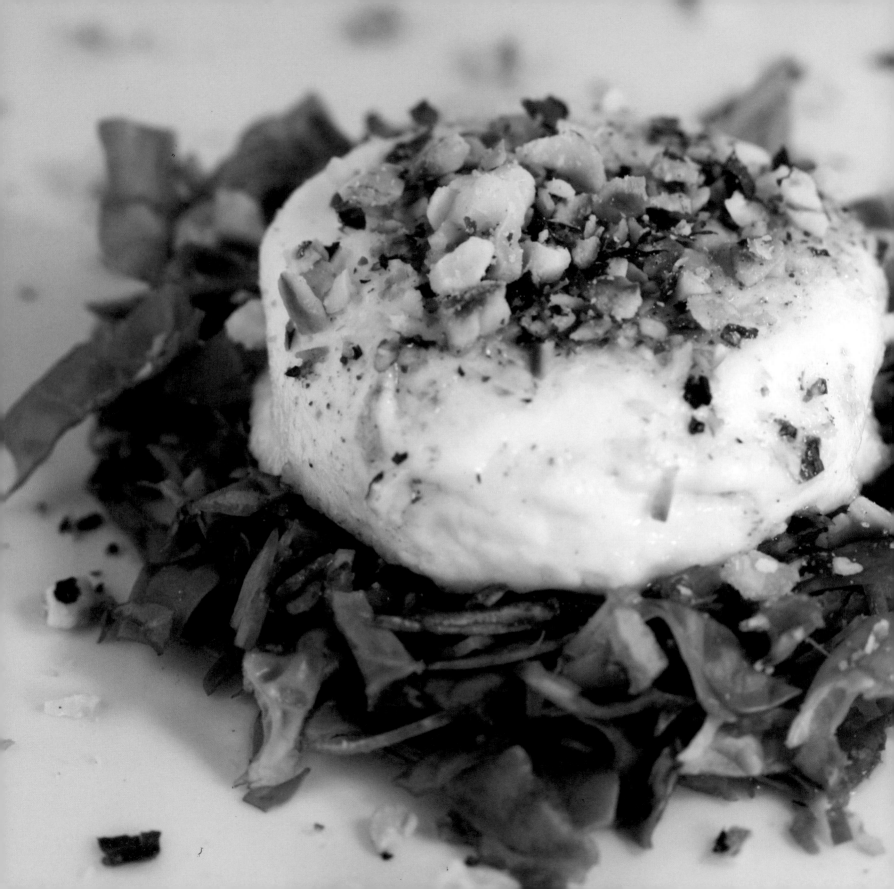

Goat's Cheese with Hazelnuts

Serves: 4
Preparation time: 5 minutes
Cooking time: 2 – 3 minutes

Ingredients:
1 Tbsp hazelnuts, roughly ground
juice of 1 lemon
¼ tsp paprika
¼ tsp ground coriander
salt and pepper
160g goat's cheese, preferably moulded as it holds together better
when cooked.
1 tsp ghee or Gabriel friendly oil (see page 24)
baby spinach leaves, cut into strips to serve

Method:
1. Place ground hazelnuts in a frying pan over medium heat. Toast lightly for 1-2 minutes. Remove from pan and set aside.
2. In a small jug combine lemon juice, paprika and coriander.
3. Place the cooking oil in a frying pan on medium to high heat. Once the oil is hot, add the goat's cheese to the pan. Cook on each side for 1-2 minutes.
4. On your serving plates, make a bed of the baby spinach leaves. Lift cheese out of the pan and place onto the bed of spinach.
5. Pour the lemon juice mixture over the top and sprinkle with the ground hazelnuts.

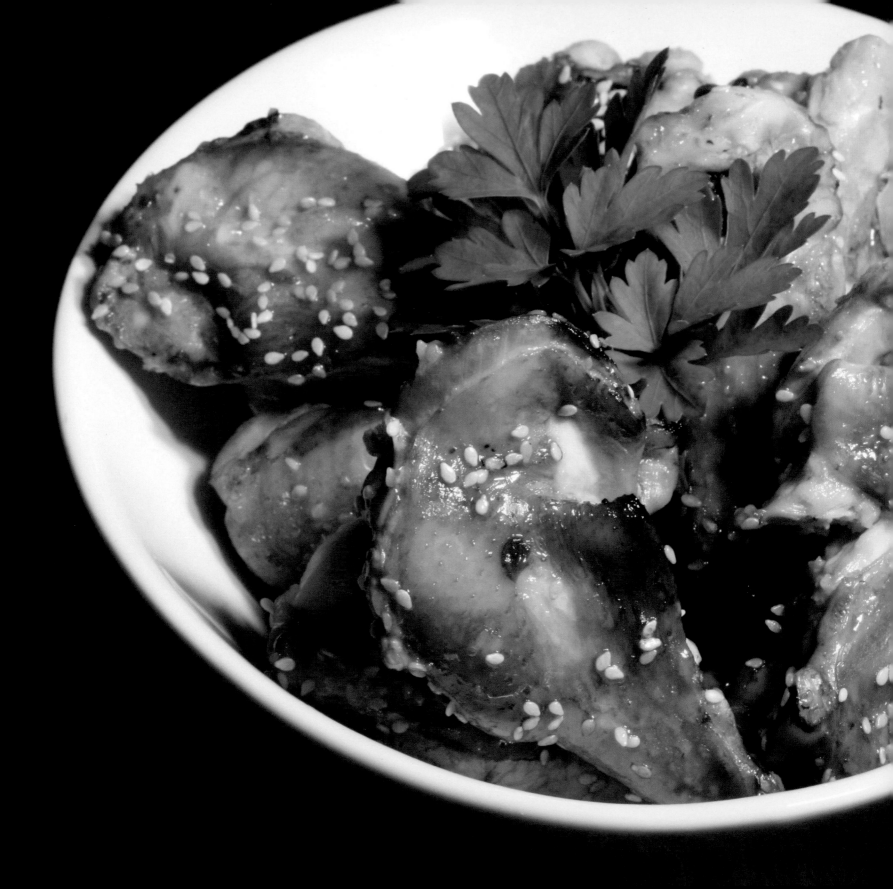

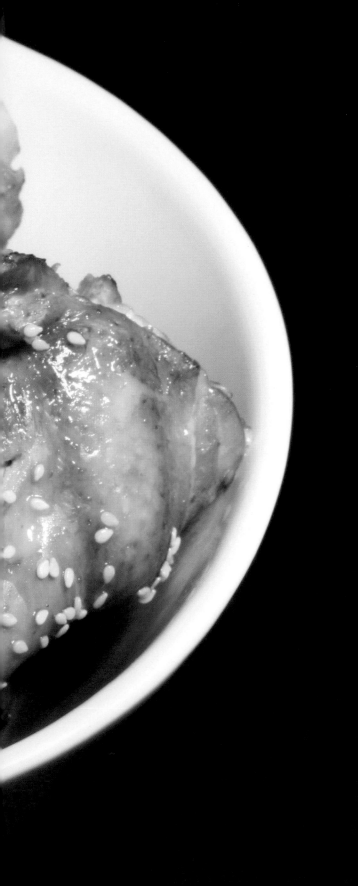

Marinated Chicken Wings

Preparation time: 10 minutes + 2 hours marinating
Cooking time: 60 minutes

Ingredients:
12 chicken wings
2 ½ Tbsp tamari
2 tsp coconut palm sugar
1 tsp xylitol
¼ cup orange juice
1 Tbsp sesame oil
1 Tbsp sesame seeds

Method:
1. In a large mixing bowl, combine tamari, coconut palm sugar, xylitol, orange juice and sesame oil. Mix together well.
2. Place the wings into the tamari mixture ensuring that each wing is coated in the marinade. Cover and refrigerate for 2 hours.
3. Preheat oven to 180°C / 355°F.
4. Pour entire contents of bowl – chicken wings and marinade – into a large baking tray. There should be enough room so that wings are not on top of each other. Sprinkle 2 teaspoons of sesame seeds over chicken.
5. Bake in oven on 180°C / 355°F for 30 minutes. Remove from oven and turn each chicken wing over. Sprinkle remaining sesame seeds over chicken. Return to oven and bake for a further 30 minutes or until cooked through.

Lunches and Dinners

These days there simply isn't enough time to spend hours in the kitchen. Lunches and dinners don't have to be complicated or difficult to prepare in order to be delicious and satisfying. With The Gabriel Method, as long as the meals contain the big three, they have all that is necessary to be complete meals in themselves.

So, even though the lunch and dinner recipes here are protein rich, we strongly recommend that they be eaten with salads and a healthy dressing to provide the live food nutrition that helps balance the whole meal.

You may find that the later meals of the day are smaller because your body has been satisfyingly nourished from an optimal breakfast. Nevertheless, the size of your lunches and dinners is up to you. Feeling deprived is just another form of starvation and will keep the FAT programs turned on. Eat as much as you want, but do it slowly and consciously, savouring as much as you can. This will give your body a chance to send the appropriate 'I'm full' signals while, at the same time, increasing your appreciation of all the sensuousness that food has to offer. Eating slowly also has the added benefit of helping your digestion, as thorough chewing makes the nutrients more easily absorbed by your digestive system.

All the lunches and dinners that we've created for you here are easy to prepare and delicious, even if we do say so ourselves!

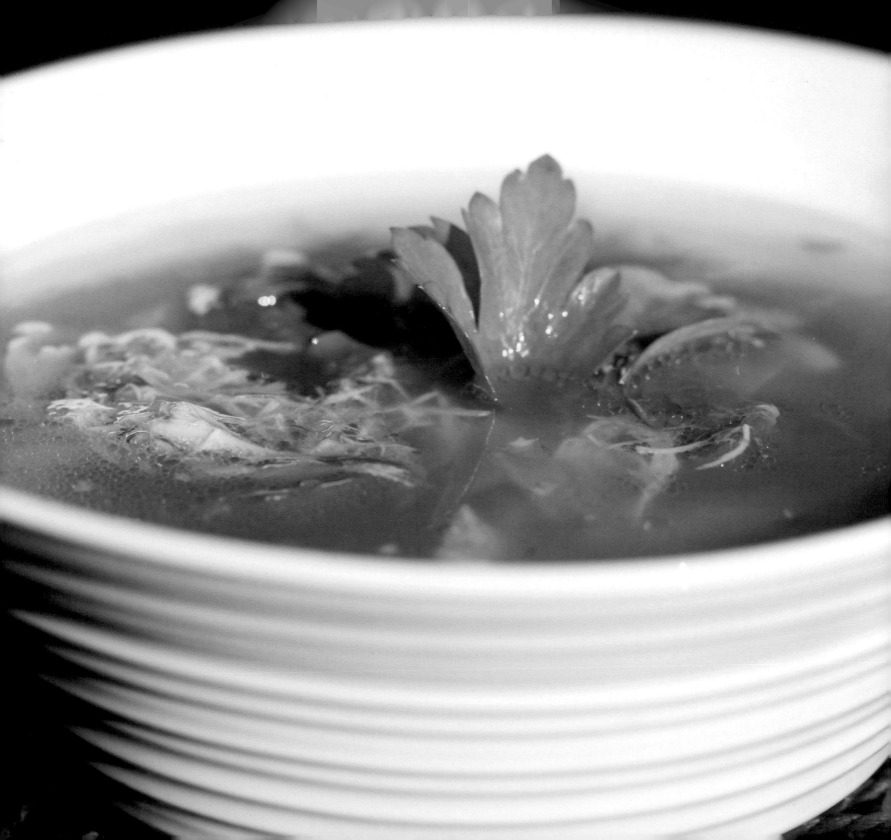

Lunches and Dinners

Prawn Laksa

Serves: 4
Preparation time: 10 minutes
Cooking time: 10 minutes

Ingredients:
1 Tbsp sesame oil
3 Tbsp laksa paste (preferably with no artificial colours or flavours)
270ml coconut milk
½ Tbsp xylitol
1 Tbsp lime juice
750g green king prawns (shrimp), peeled
2cm fresh ginger
4 baby pak choy, trimmed, leaves separated
½ cup fresh mint
½ cup bean sprouts
2 cups of water

Method:
1. Heat oil in a wok or large frying pan on medium heat. Add laksa paste cooking until the fragrance becomes apparent. Add water, coconut milk, xylitol and lime juice.
2. Increase the heat to high. Bring contents of frying pan to the boil. Add prawns (shrimp) and ginger.
3. Reduce heat to low-medium. Simmer until colour of prawns changes to pink.
4. Add pak choy and simmer for 1 more minute before serving.
5. Serve topped with bean sprouts, fresh mint and extra lime wedges.

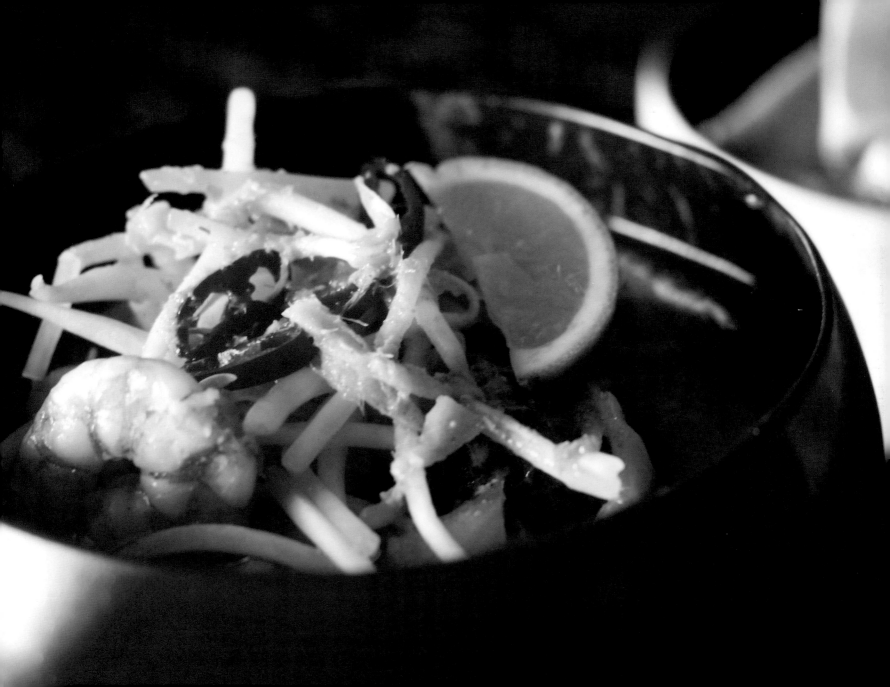

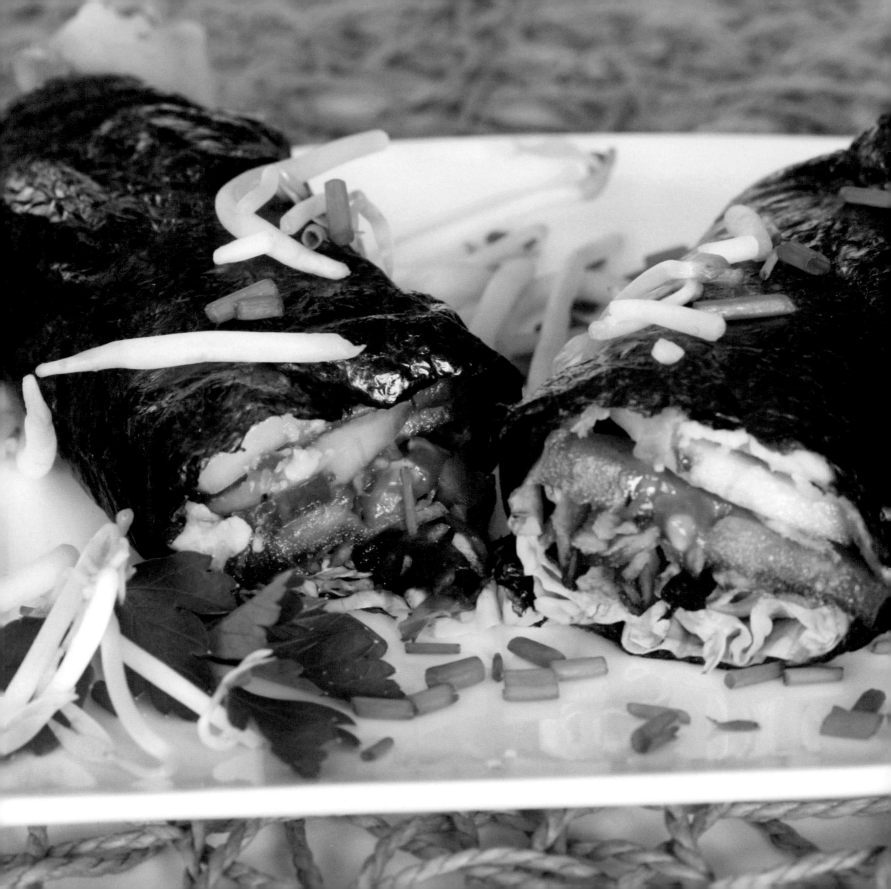

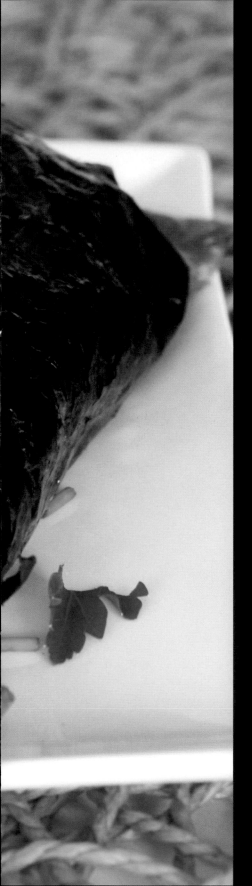

Nori Wraps

Serves: 2
Preparation time: 10 minutes

Ingredients:

2 fresh nori sheets
½ avocado, sliced thinly
1 carrot, grated
1 small beetroot, grated

½ cucumber, sliced
100g smoked salmon
1 tomato, sliced thinly
1 Tbsp flax seeds, ground
lettuce leaves, washed and spun

Method:

1. Place nori sheet on chopping board, shiny side down.
2. Layer your choice of favourite fillings on top of each other, leaving about 1 inch of nori sheet clear at the end closest to you.
3. Gently roll the front of the nori sheet over fillings and continue to roll gently to the end. If you are having trouble getting the paper to stick to itself, dip your fingers in warm water and spread along seam.
4. Cut into 2 pieces to make for easy eating. Enjoy!

Other Gabrielicious favourite fillings:

haloumi
wasabi
pickled ginger

tuna
sprouts
smoked chicken

A great alternative to the traditional wrap or even sandwiches. Seaweed is loaded with trace minerals and very assimilable calcium. I am often grateful at lunch time when Jenny, my office manager, prepares one of these for me. Thanks Jen!

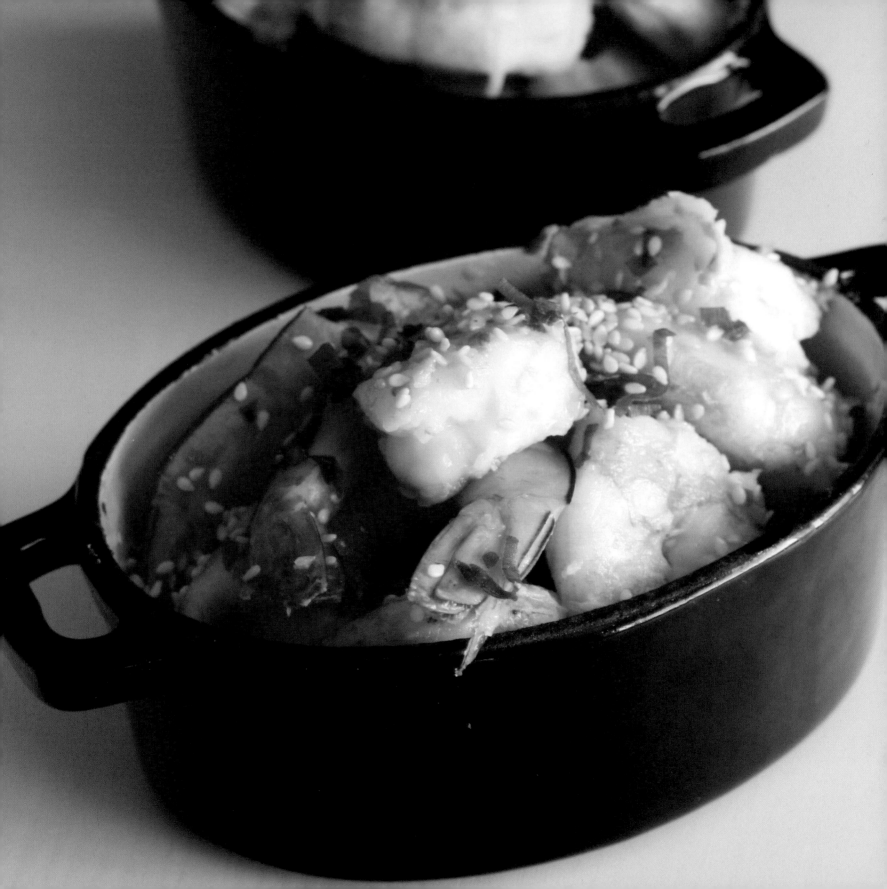

Sesame Garlic Prawns (shrimp)

Serves: 4
Preparation time: 5 minutes + 30 minutes marinating time
Cooking time: 3 minutes

Ingredients:
20 prawns (shrimp), peeled
2 Tbsp sesame oil
4 cloves of garlic, crushed
1 Tbsp ghee
2 Tbsp sesame seeds
1 Tbsp flax seeds
1 lime, cut into wedges

Method:
1. Place sesame oil, garlic and prawns (shrimp) in medium sized bowl. Cover and refrigerate for 30 minutes.
2. Melt ghee in frying pan on medium to high heat. Add prawns (shrimp) to pan and cook for approximately 3 minutes or until prawns begin to change colour.
3. Serve sprinkled with sesame seeds, flax seeds and a squeeze of lime juice.

Chilli

Serves: 4
Preparation time: 10 minutes
Cooking time: 15 minutes

Ingredients:
1 Tbsp Gabriel friendly cooking oil (see page 24)
1 onion, sliced
500g mince meat
1 medium green capsicum (bell pepper), cut into small pieces
4 tomatoes, crushed or 1 tin tomatoes
2 Tbsp tomato paste
1 clove garlic, peeled and crushed
½ lemon, juiced
½ tsp cumin
¼ cup red wine
½ tsp chilli or to your liking, optional
cheese, grated to serve

Method:
1. Heat cooking oil in pan. Add onion and cook until lightly browned. Add mince meat. Stir in pan to separate meat.
2. Add capsicum (bell pepper), tomatoes, tomato paste and garlic. Stir to combine. Cook until meat is cooked through.
3. Add lemon juice, wine, cumin and chilli powder. Stir to combine.
4. Season with salt and pepper. Serve with grated cheese.

"Here's to you, Dad!
For all those memories warming
up after hours on the slopes."

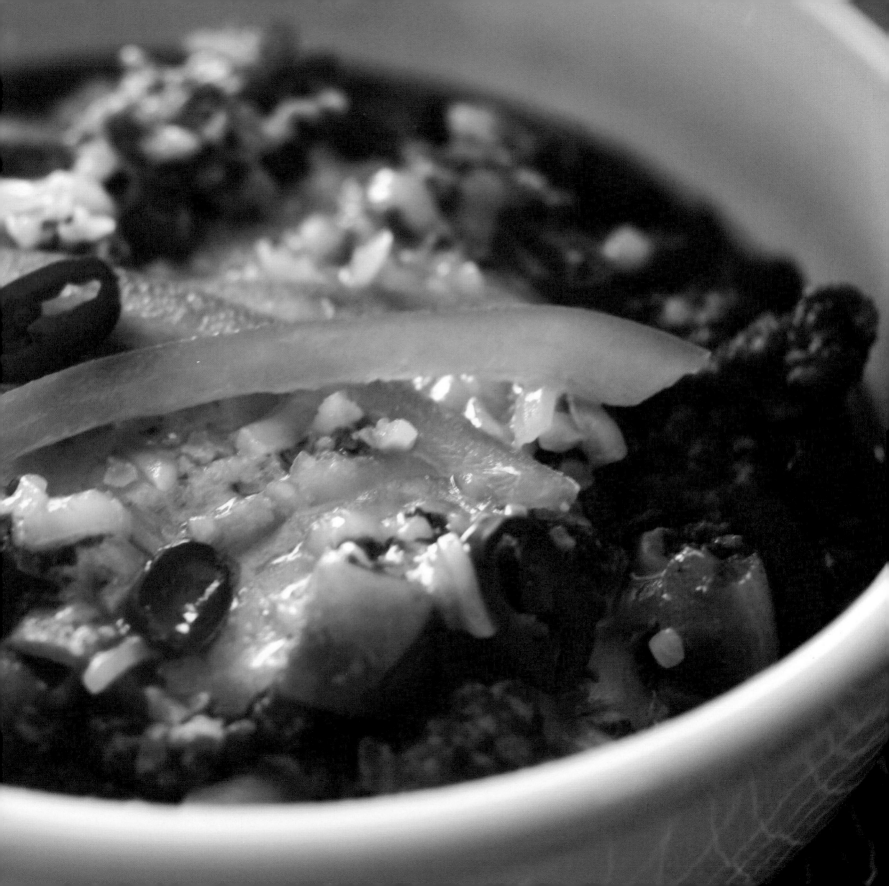

Mushroom and Spinach Egg Roll

Serves: 2
Preparation time: 15 minutes
Cooking time: 10 minutes

Ingredients:
4 eggs (organic, free range) + 2 extra egg yolks
1 Tbsp Ghee or Gabriel friendly cooking oil (see page 24)
3 large mushrooms, sliced
1 Tbsp tamari
1 clove garlic (optional), crushed
handful of baby spinach

Method:
1. Beat eggs and egg yolks together in bowl.
2. Melt 1 Tbsp ghee in frying pan on medium heat.
3. Cook mushrooms in frying pan stirring as you add tamari and garlic. Take out of pan after 2-3 minutes or after mushrooms are cooked and set aside. Cover them to keep warm.
4. Melt the rest of ghee in frying pan. Place beaten eggs in pan so that mixture is well distributed. Cook until you can slide a spatula underneath the omelette.
5. Slide omelette out of pan onto flat chopping board, or other flat surface.
6. Place spinach leaves and mushrooms at one end of omelette. Roll omelette up keeping as tight as possible.
7. To serve either cut in half or cut into 2.5cm slices. Place a toothpick into roll and serve as finger food.

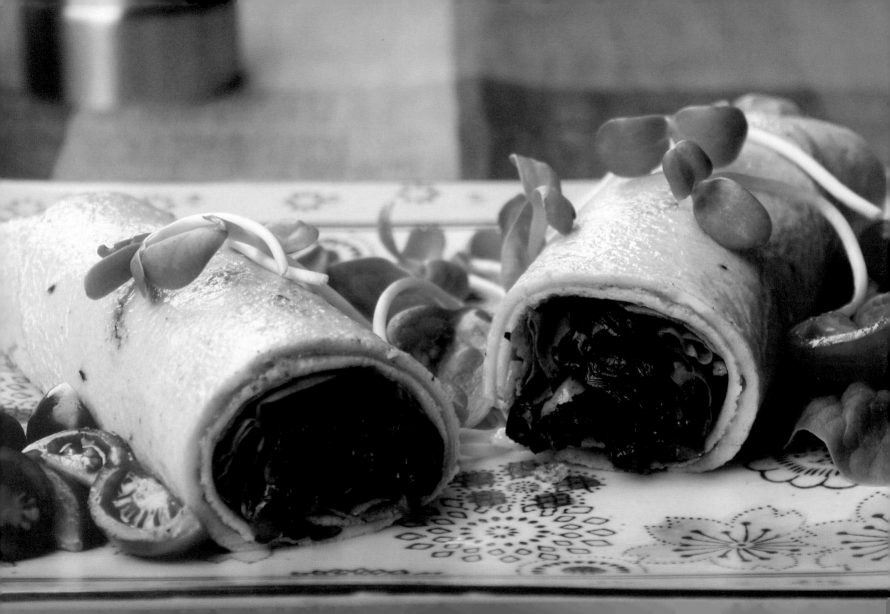

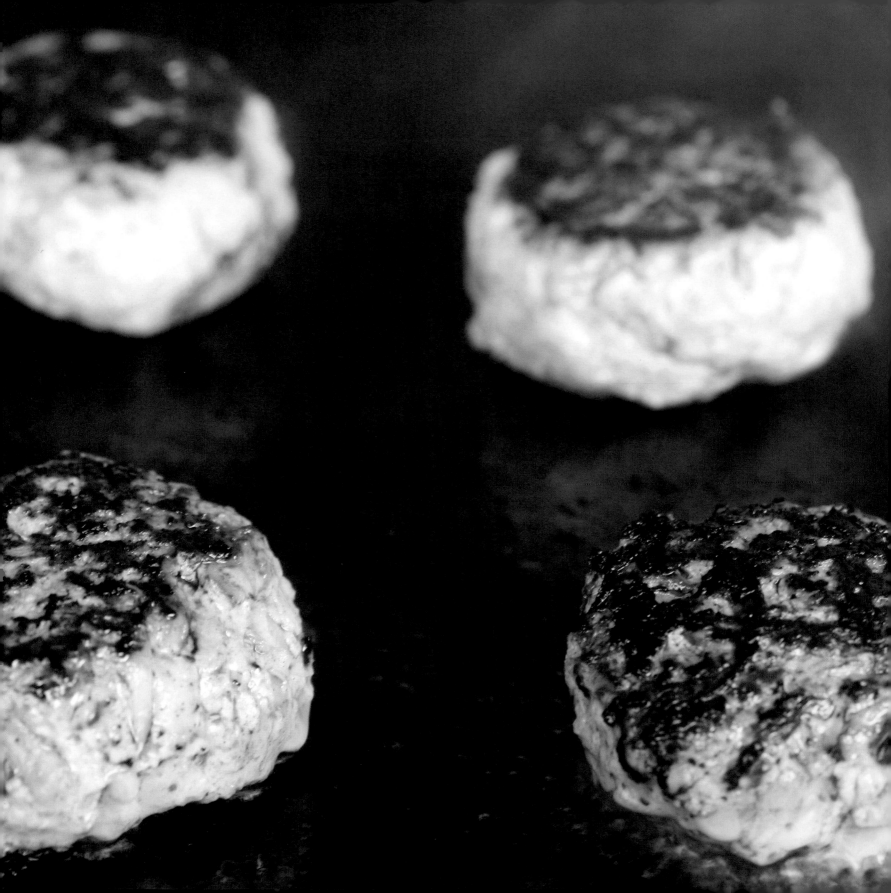

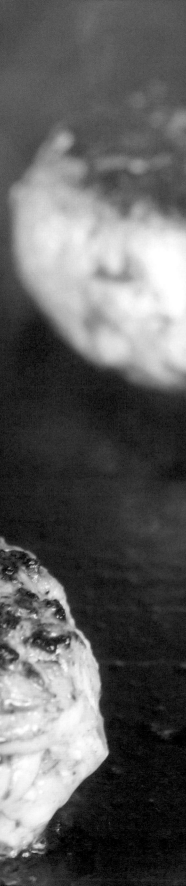

Onionless Rissoles

Serves: 14
Preparation time: 10 minutes
Cooking time: 15 minutes

Ingredients:
500g mince beef (organic grass-fed)
100g grated zucchini (approximately ½ a zucchini)
3 cloves garlic, crushed
1 Tbsp oregano leaves
1 egg yolk
healthy salt (see page 17) and pepper
1 Tbsp Gabriel Method cooking oil (see page 24)

Method:
1. Combine all ingredients together in a bowl.
2. Make patties that fit into the palm of your hand (approximately 2 tablespoons) and place on clean plate. You can refrigerate these until time to cook, this will also help them set.
3. Melt 1 tablespoon ghee in frying pan or BBQ and cook rissoles on medium heat until browned. Turn and cook until browned on second side and cooked through.
4. Serve with salad sprinkled with flax seeds.

Jon's translation of rissoles: an Australian meat dish half-way between a meatloaf and a hamburger.

Especially for our favourite little onion-disliking man. Xabi, these are for you!
– Feel free to add onions if you prefer - Oona

119

Bubbe's Chicken Soup

Serves: 8
Preparation time: 15 minutes
Cooking time: 1.5 hours

Ingredients:

1 whole chicken (organic, free range), washed
2 onions, quartered
3 cloves garlic, peeled and crushed
4 carrots, sliced in rounds
½ bunch celery, sliced
2 Tbsp dill, cut finely
½ cup parsley, chopped finely
healthy salt (see page 17) and pepper to taste
2 chicken stock cubes, MSG Free

Method:

1. Place chicken in large saucepan. Cover with water and place on stove top on high heat. Allow water to boil. Cook for 1 hour.
2. Using a slotted spoon, remove chicken from pot, preserving stock. Place chicken on large plate or baking dish. Separate meat from bones. Return meat to pot and discard bones.
3. Add remaining ingredients to pan. Allow to cook for another 20 minutes.
4. Serve garnished with fresh dill or parsley.

*"Your one pot, get-well soup nurtures body, belly, taste buds and heart.
The Gabriel Method's adaptation of my mum's home made chicken soup, always made and served with so much love."*

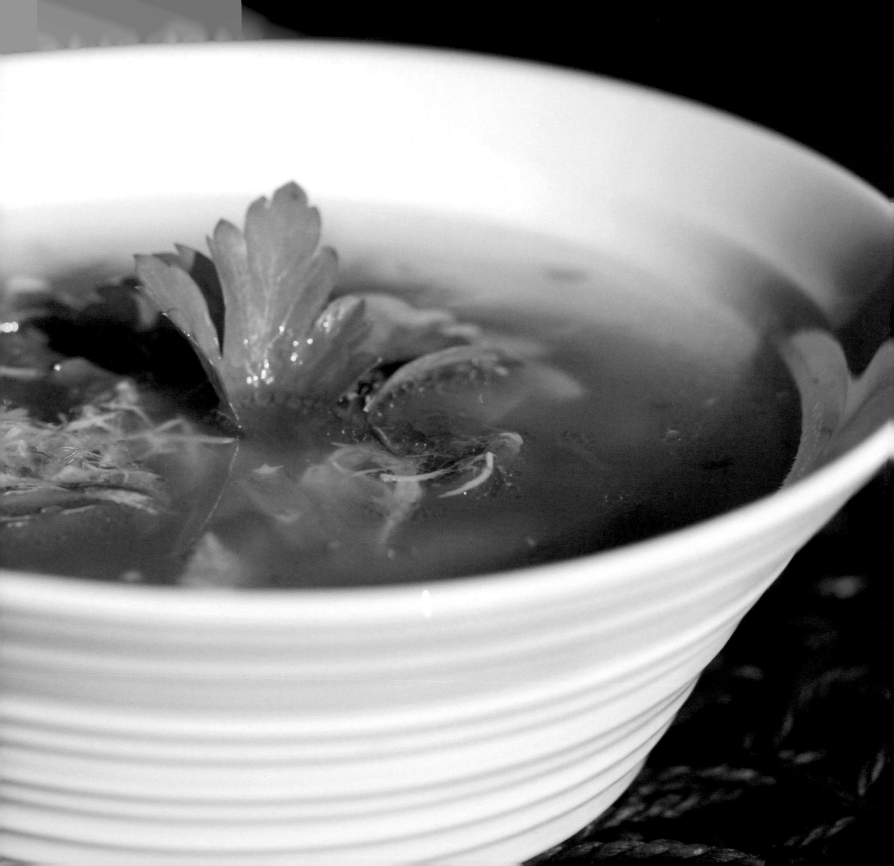

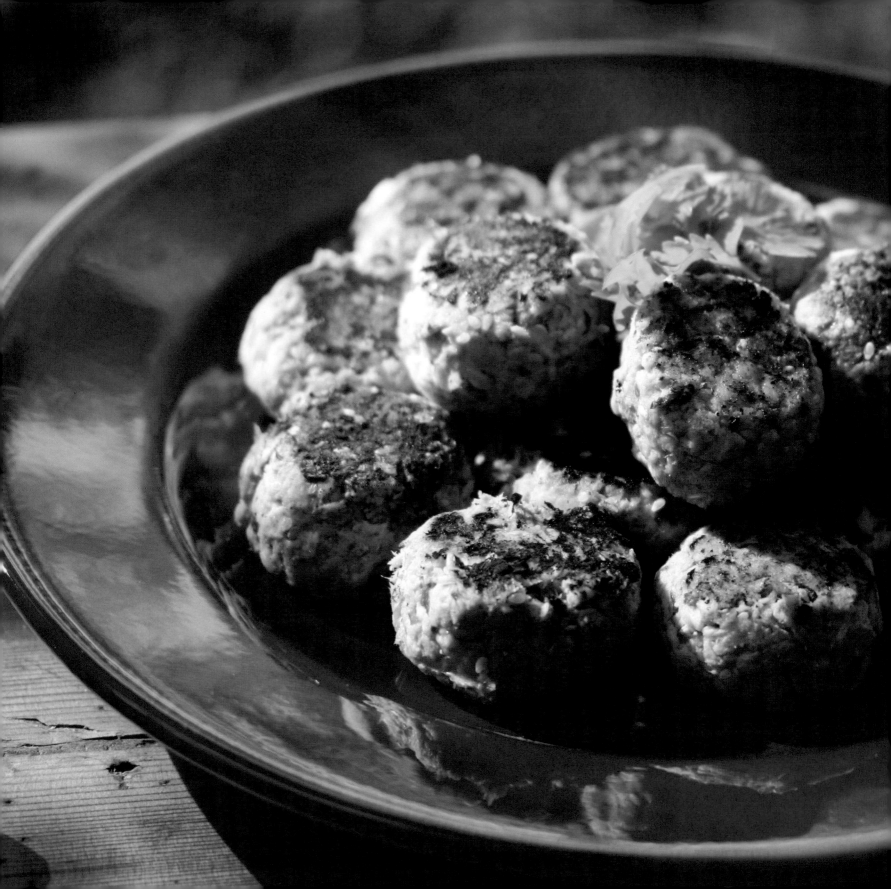

Fish Cakes

Serves: 12
Preparation time: 15 minutes
Cooking time: 15 minutes

Ingredients:
500g white flesh fish fillets, already cooked
2 Tbsp lime juice
1 Tbsp ground coriander
½ cup fresh coriander, cut finely
2 Tbsp sesame seeds
2 Tbsp organic coconut cream
1 Tbsp red curry paste
3 spring onions (scallions), sliced
1 egg yolk
1 Tbsp ghee or Gabriel Method cooking oil
(see page 24)

Method:
1. Cut cooked fish into small pieces. Crumble fish with your fingers to break it up into small pieces. Add all the other ingredients and stir well to combine.
2. Shape into patties, approximately 2 tablespoons each. Place on a clean plate until ready to cook.
3. Heat cooking oil in frying pan or BBQ and cook fish cakes on medium heat until browned. Turn and cook until browned on second side and cooked through.
4. Serve with salad sprinkled with flax seeds.

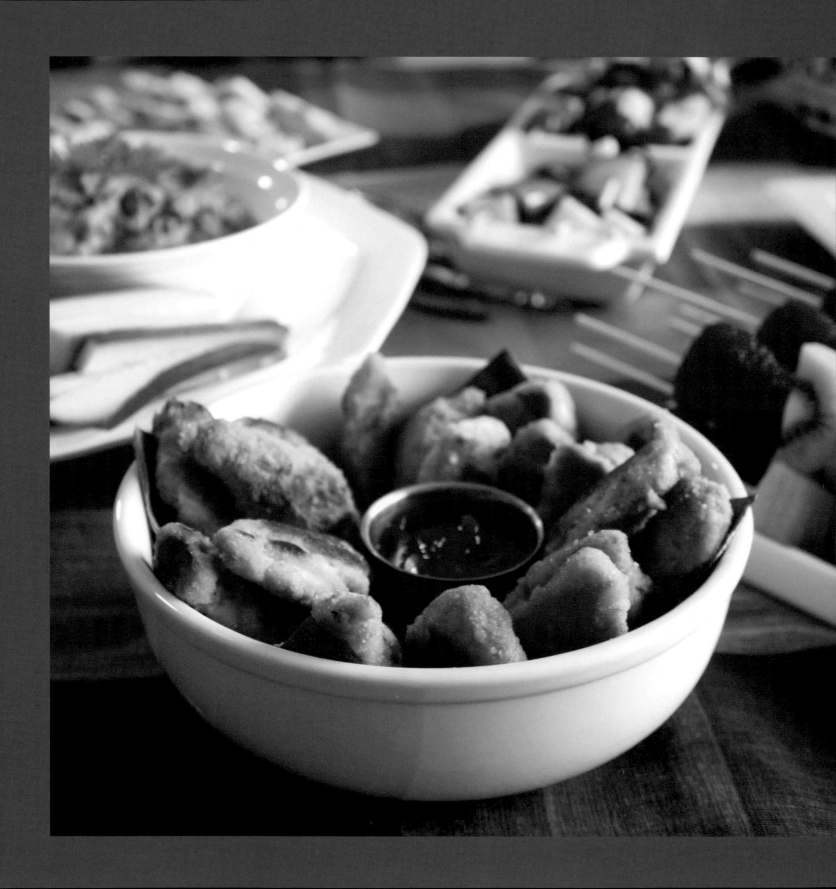

Chicken Nuggets

Serves: 4
Preparation time: 15 minutes
Cooking time: 20 minutes

Ingredients:
4 chicken thigh fillets (organic, free range), cut into nuggets
2 egg yolks, beaten
½ cup organic ground almonds
1 Tbsp ghee for cooking

Method:
1. Place beaten egg yolks in one bowl and place ground almonds in a second bowl.
2. Dip each chicken piece into egg yolk mix and then into ground almonds so that it is coated in almonds. Place coated chicken pieces onto plate.
3. Melt ghee in frying pan on medium heat. When it is hot place chicken into pan. Cook on each side for 2-3 minutes or until almonds are golden brown and chicken cooked through. Do this in batches until all chicken pieces are cooked.
4. Serve with Gabriel Method Tomato Sauce (see page 206).

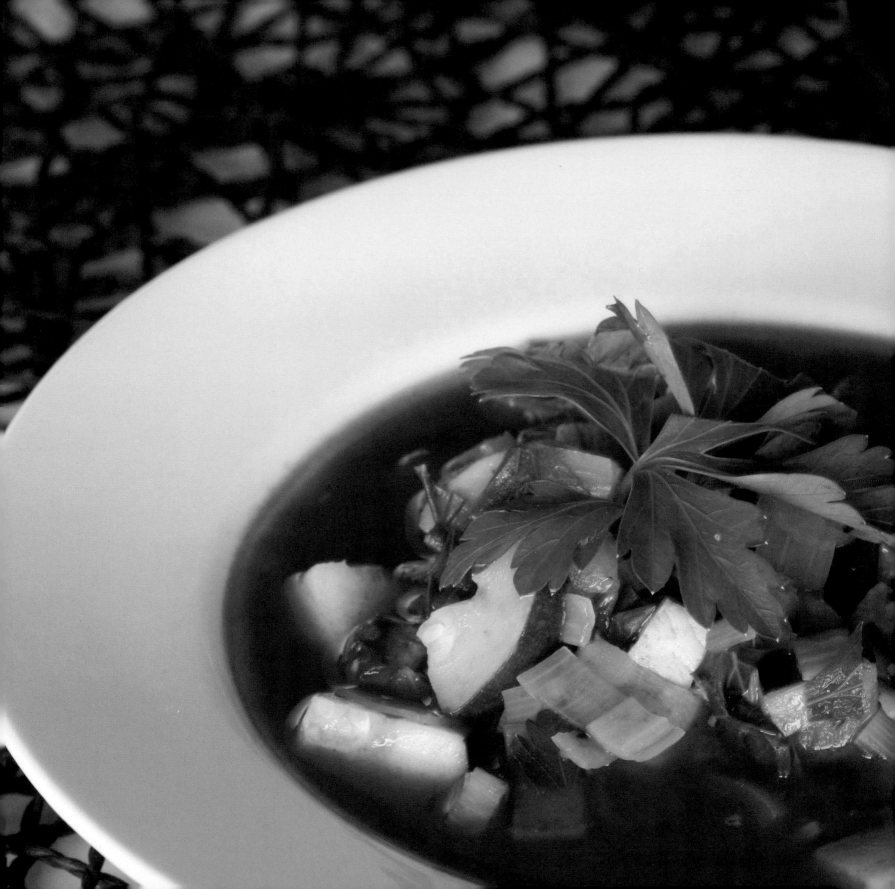

Hammed Up Minestrone

Serves: 6
Preparation time: 30 minutes
Cooking time: 30 minutes

Ingredients:
1 Tbsp Ghee of Gabriel friendly cooking oil (see page 24)
1 slice thickly sliced smoked ham (organic, free range), cubed
1 onion, sliced
1 leek, sliced
3 cloves garlic, crushed
4 cups water
2 cups fresh tomatoes, crushed or 1 tin crushed tomatoes
2 Tbsp tomato paste
2 carrots, peeled and cubed
1 zucchini, sliced into quarter rounds
½ cup fresh basil, coarsely chopped
2 bay leaves
1 cup Parmesan cheese, grated
healthy salt (see page 17) and pepper

Method:
1. In a large soup pot, heat oil. Fry cubed ham until beginning to brown.
2. Add onion, leek and garlic and cook for a further 6-8 minutes or until softened.
3. Add 4 cups of water. Cover pot and boil.
4. Add tomatoes, tomato paste, carrots, zucchini, basil and bay leaves. Simmer for 20-30 minutes or until vegetables are tender.
5. Add Parmesan cheese. Cook for a further 5 minutes until cheese has melted through.
6. Season with healthy salt and pepper to taste.

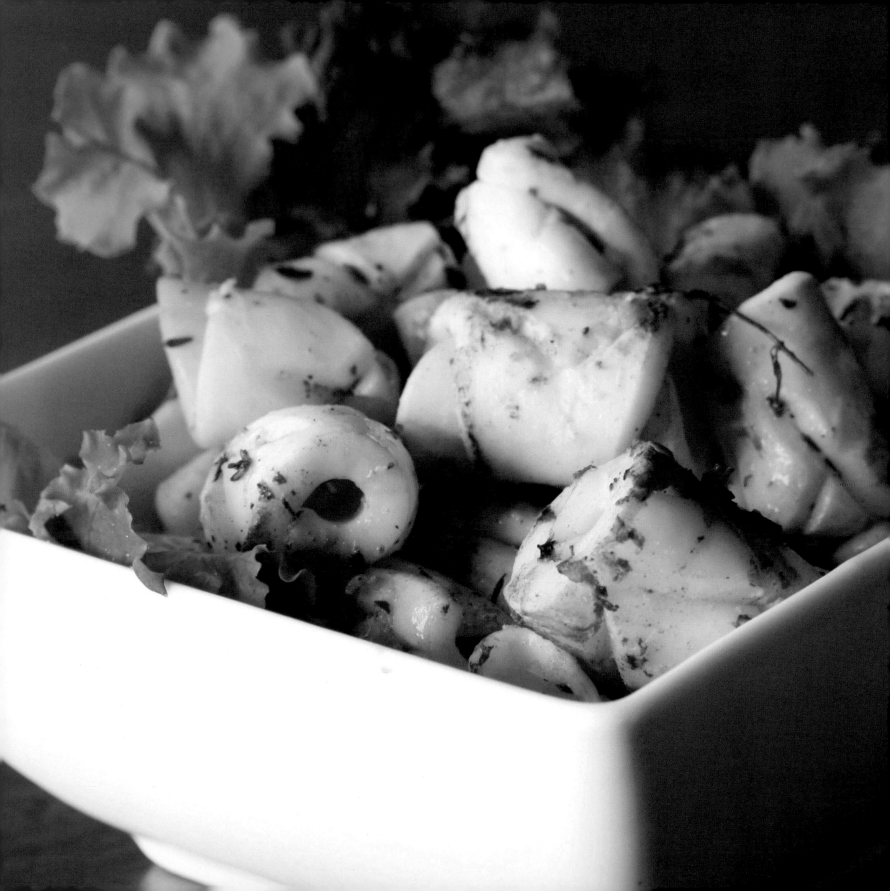

BBQ'd Lemon and Thyme Calamari

Preparation time: 20 minutes plus 1 hour marinating
Cooking time: 15 minutes

Ingredients:
1kg (about 12) small, cleaned calamari tubes (hoods)
olive oil, to grease

Marinade:
juice of 3 lemons
¼ cup of olive oil
2 Tbsp fresh thyme leaves
1 large fresh red chillies, deseeded,
finely chopped
1 tsp sesame oil
healthy salt (see page 17) & freshly
ground black pepper
lettuce leaves to serve
lemon wedges to serve

Method:
1. To make the marinade, combine the lemon juice, olive oil, thyme and chillies in a large airtight container. Season with salt and pepper.
2. Cut each calamari tube into quarters lengthways. Score the inside surface of each in a diamond pattern (don't cut all the way through). Cut each quarter into 3 even pieces. Add the calamari to the marinade and toss to coat. Place in the fridge for 1 hour to marinate (or longer if time permits).
3. Brush a barbecue plate with oil to grease and preheat on high. Spoon half the calamari and marinade onto preheated barbecue and cook for 1-2 minutes each side or until calamari curls and is opaque. Transfer to a bowl and cover to keep warm. Repeat with remaining calamari and marinade.
4. Place calamari and any juices in a large serving bowl. Season with salt and pepper, and toss gently to combine. Serve immediately.

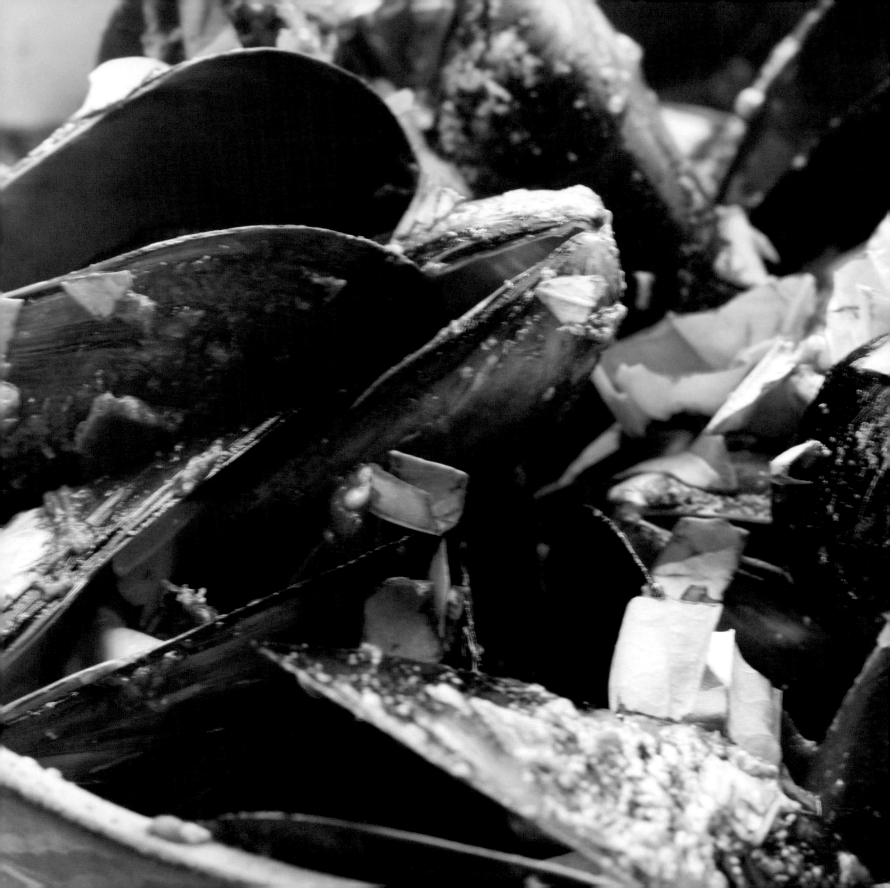

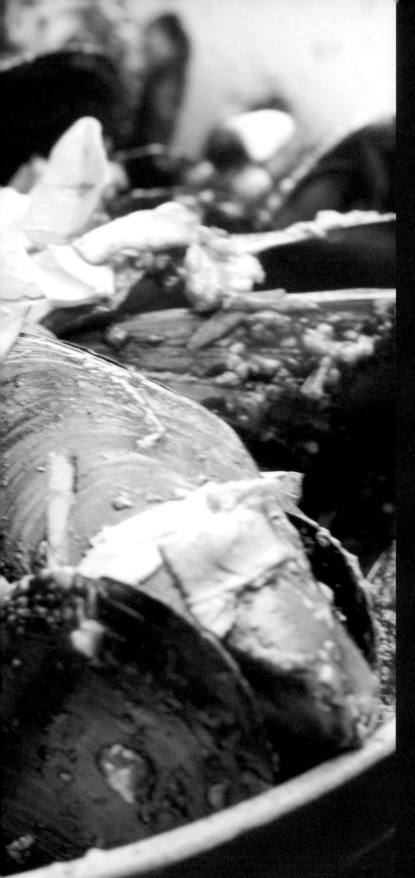

Chilli Mussels

Serves: 4
Preparation time: 10 minutes
Cooking time: 10 minutes

Ingredients:

1 kg mussels
1 Tbsp Gabriel friendly cooking oil (see page 24)
1 brown onion, diced
1 garlic clove, peeled and crushed
2 cups tomatoes, puréed in food processor
1 tsp chilli powder OR fresh chilli*
½ cup fresh basil leaves, finely shredded

*Adjust quantities of chilli to suit personal taste.
This recipe will make for a very mild chilli sauce.

Method:

1. Rinse and debeard all mussels. Discard any open mussels that do not close when held under running water while applying pressure. Set aside.
2. Heat cooking oil in medium saucepan on medium heat.
3. Cook onion in saucepan until beginning to colour. Add garlic and allow to cook for one minute. Add puréed tomatoes and chilli powder. Stir until sauce is well heated.
4. Remove sauce from heat.
5. Place the mussels in a large, empty pot with lid on high heat.
6. Heat for approximately 5 minutes or until all mussels are open.
7. Place mussels in a large serving bowl or individual serving bowls. Distribute sauce over mussels. Stir sauce and mussels together and sprinkle with shredded basil leaves prior to serving.

Home-Made Dukkah

Makes: 1 cup
Preparation time: 5 minutes
Cooking time: 10 minutes

Ingredients:

⅓ cup hazelnuts
¼ cup sesame seeds
2 tsp coriander, ground

2 tsp cumin, ground
salt and pepper to taste

Method:

1. Place hazelnuts in a dry frying pan on medium – high heat. Cook, stirring from time to time, for approximately 5 minutes or until toasted. Grind hazelnuts using a coffee grinder or small food processor.
2. Toast sesame seeds in frying pan for 2-3 minutes. Add remaining ingredients and cook for approximately 30 seconds.
3. Combine sesame seed mixture and ground hazelnuts together in a bowl.

Dukkah Chicken Bites

Serves: 4
Preparation time: 15 minutes
Cooking time: 20 minutes

Ingredients:
4 chicken thigh fillets (organic, free range), cut into long strips
2 egg yolks, beaten
1 cup dukkah mix*
2-3 Tbsp Gabriel friendly cooking oil (see page 24)

*If you don't want to make your own, dukkah can be purchased from most supermarkets, delis and gourmet food shops

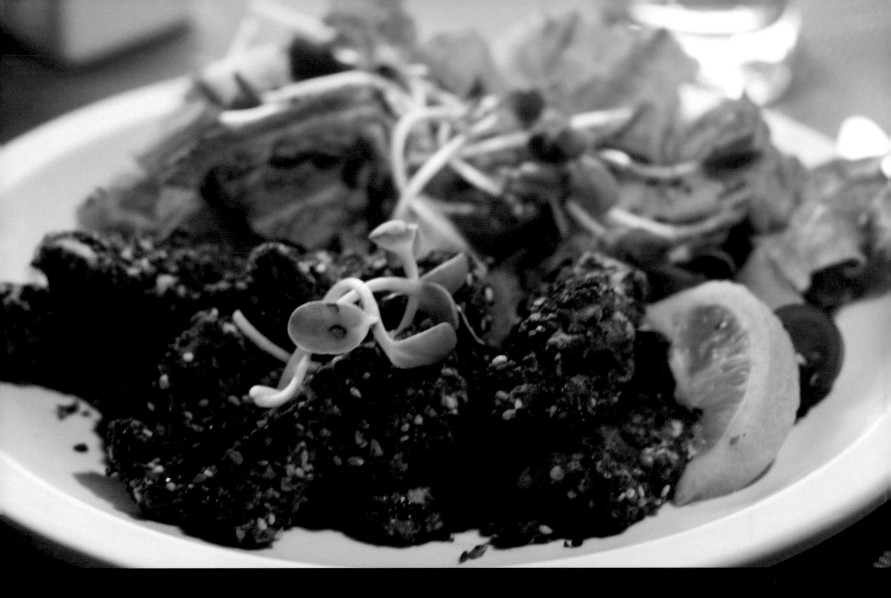

Method:
1. Have beaten eggs yolks in one bowl and dukkah in a second bowl.
2. Dip each chicken piece into egg yolk mix and then into dukkah so that it is coated all over. Place coated chicken pieces onto a plate.
3. Heat 1 Tbsp cooking oil in frying pan on medium – high heat. When it is hot, place chicken into pan. Cook on each side for 2-3 minutes or until chicken is cooked through.

Omelette Pizza

Makes: 1 Pizza
Preparation time: 15 minutes
Cooking time: 20 minutes

Ingredients:
1 Tbsp Gabriel friendly cooking oil (see page 24)
4 eggs (organic, free range), beaten
2 Tbsp tomato pizza sauce
8 baby spinach leaves
¼ onion, sliced thinly
1 mushroom, sliced thinly
¼ cup cheddar cheese, grated
¼ cup mozzarella, grated

Method:
1. Heat cooking oil in medium sized frying pan on medium heat.
2. Pour beaten eggs into pan. Swirl the pan around so that egg is evenly distributed.
3. Allow to cook for one minute or until you can see that the underside is cooked. Reduce heat and flip omelette over to cook second side. Take caution when doing this so that you don't break the omelette. Cook for another minute or until cooked through.
4. Remove omelette and place onto plate or wooden chopping board.
5. Spread tomato sauce evenly over omelette. Add spinach leaves, mushroom, onion slices and cheeses.
6. Place prepared omelette pizza under medium grill for a few minutes until cheese has browned.

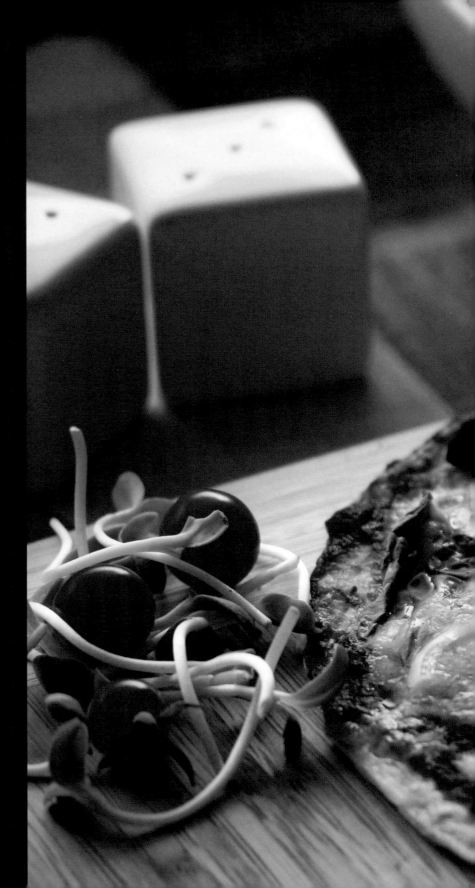

By using an egg base you are getting protein into your meal rather than dead carbs, with no taste sacrificed. The key to good pizza is in the sauce. You use such a small amount and it can make or break the whole pizza experience. If you've got a great homemade pizza sauce go for it, but otherwise, this is one of the rare instances where I actually recommend getting a store bought sauce. For some reason, store-bought pizza sauces just taste more like pizza to me.

There are many good ones on the market. Where possible choose one which has organic tomatoes, no sugar or artificial sweeteners, or at the very least, no artificial colours or flavours.

The other component to a great pizza is toppings, so choose all the fresh, healthy, yummy toppings you like. Abondanza!

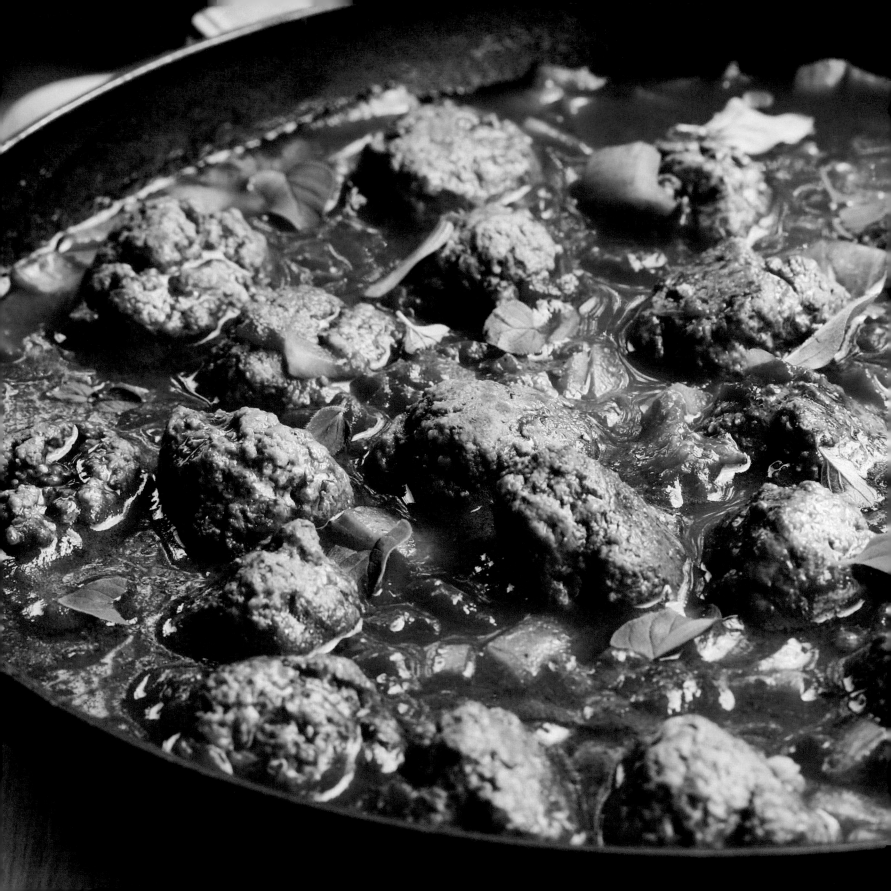

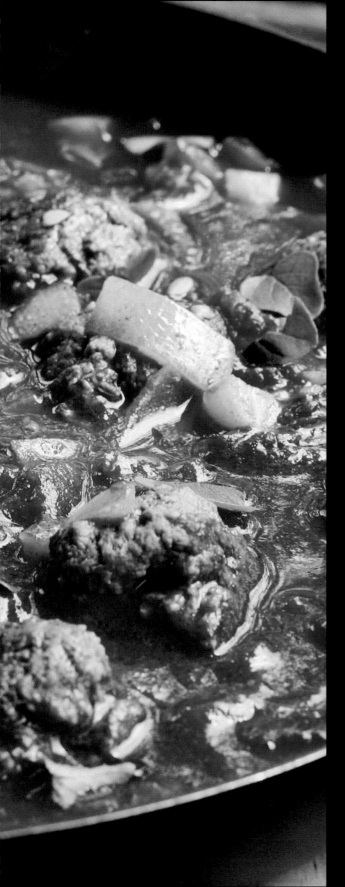

Easy Meatballs

Serves: 4
Preparation time: 20 minutes
Cooking time: 20 minutes

Ingredients for the meatballs:
500g (1lb) beef (organic grass-fed), minced (ground)
1 egg yolk (organic, free range)
healthy salt (see page 17) and pepper

Ingredients for the sauce:
1 Tbsp Gabriel friendly cooking oil (see page 24)
1 onion, diced
2 garlic cloves, finely chopped
400g (13oz) tomatoes, chopped
150ml chicken stock (with no MSG, artificial colours or flavours)
healthy salt (see page 17) and pepper

Method:
1. To make the meatballs, place beef, egg yolk and salt in a bowl and stir to combine. With wet hands, shape the meat mixture into balls. The mixture should make approximately 20 meatballs.
2. Heat cooking oil in a large frying pan. Cook meatballs in the pan over a medium to high heat, turning until browned all over. Transfer to a plate and set aside.
3. To make the sauce, add the onion to the pan and cook for approximately 5 minutes or until beginning to brown. Add the garlic, tomatoes, stock, salt and pepper. Stir the sauce while cooking. Bring the sauce to a boil.
4. Reduce the heat. Place the meatballs into the sauce and spoon the sauce over the meatballs so that they are covered. Cook for another 5 minutes or until meatballs are cooked through.

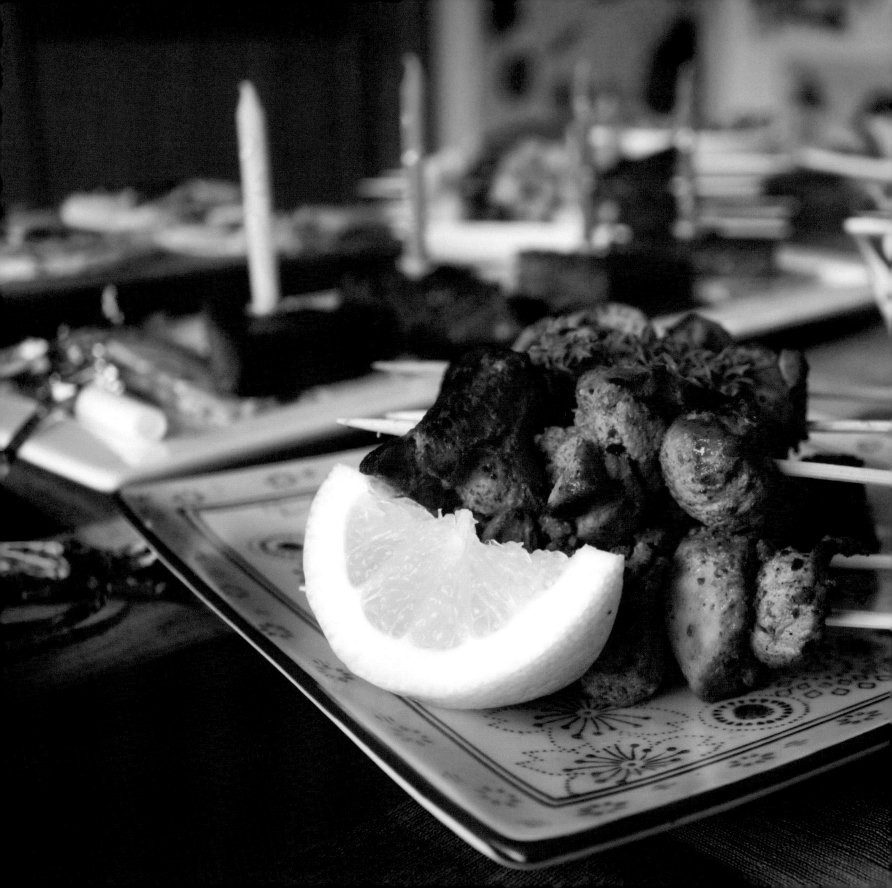

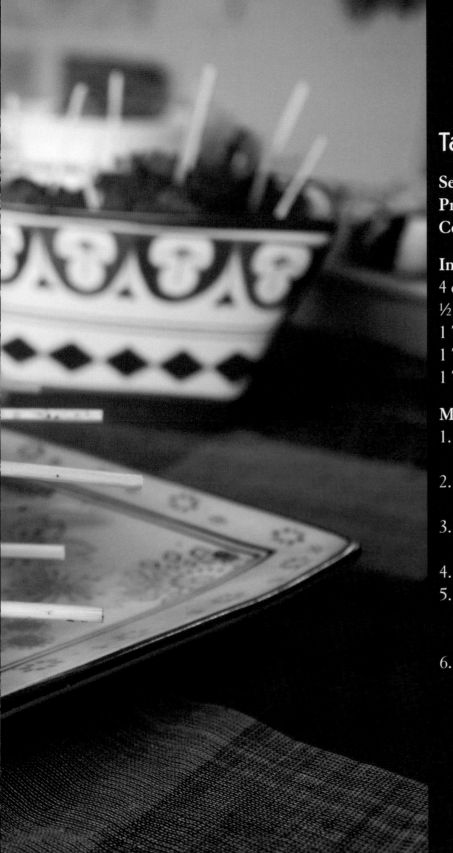

Tandoori Chicken (Kebabs)

Serves: 2
Preparation time: 10 minutes + 1 hour marinating
Cooking time: 10 minutes

Ingredients:
4 chicken thigh fillets (organic, free range) cubed
½ cup plain Greek yoghurt
1 Tbsp tandoori paste
1 Tbsp lemon juice
1 Tbsp Gabriel friendly cooking oil (see page 24)

Method:
1. For kebabs, thread chicken pieces onto skewers. Place in marinating dish.
2. Combine yoghurt, tandoori paste and lemon juice in a bowl.
3. Pour tandoori mix over chicken and ensure all chicken is covered.
4. Leave in fridge to marinate for at least 1 hour.
5. Heat 1 tablespoon cooking oil in frying pan on medium-high heat. Add chicken to pan and cook, turning regularly until chicken is cooked through.
6. Serve with delicious garden salad sprinkled with flax seeds.

Simple Chicken Stir Fry

Serves: 2
Preparation time: 15 minutes
Cooking time: 15 minutes

Ingredients:
1 Tbsp Gabriel friendly cooking oil (see page 24)
500g chicken fillets (organic, free range), cut into strips
1 onion, sliced
100g zucchini, sliced into small quarters
4 broccoli florets, sliced
1 small red capsicum (bell pepper), sliced lengthways
1 clove garlic, peeled and crushed
2 Tbsp tamari
2 Tbsp flax seeds, ground

Method:
1. Heat cooking oil in frying pan on medium heat.
2. Add chicken to pan and cook until browned all over. Remove from pan and set aside.
3. Add onion to pan. Cook, stirring, for 1 minute then add zucchini, broccoli, red capsicum and garlic. Cook, stirring, for another minute or 2 then return chicken to pan. Add tamari. Stir through. Serve hot sprinkled with flax seeds.

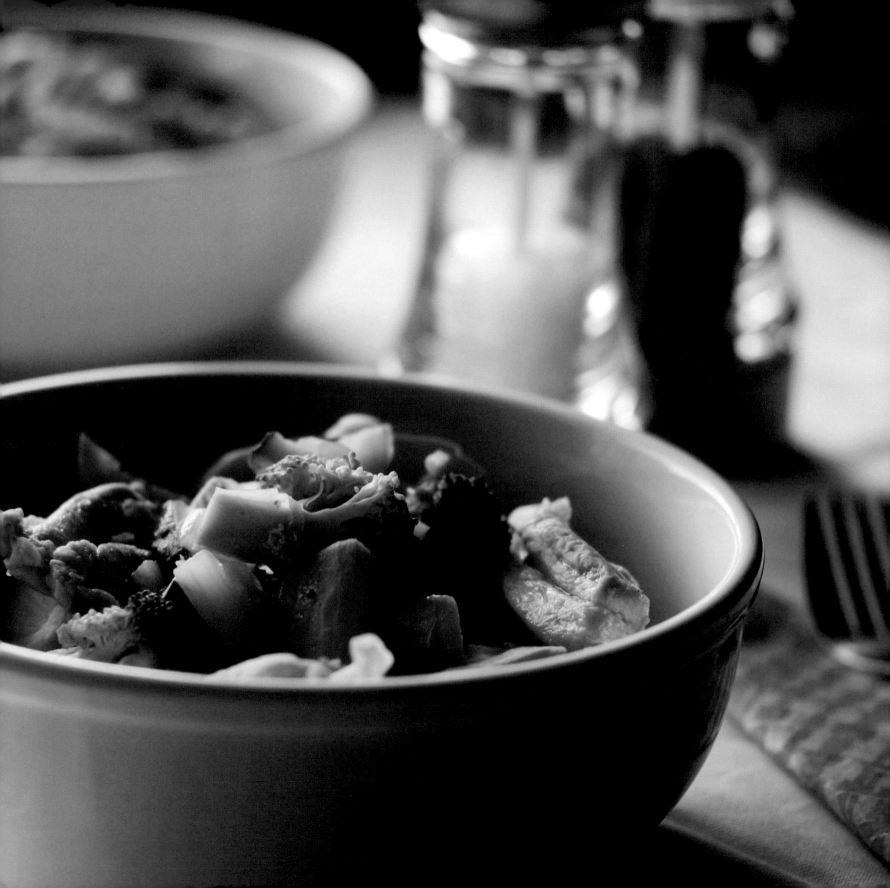

Kangaroo is a very healthy meat because it's lean and since it's wild it is guaranteed to be grass fed, and free of hormones, pesticides and grains. You can also use venison.

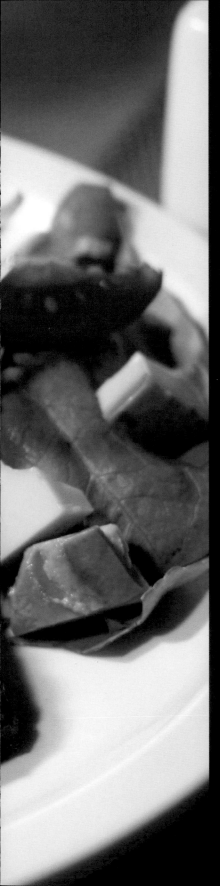

Marinated Roo Steaks

Serves: 2
Preparation time: 15 minutes
Cooking time: 10 minutes

Ingredients:
1 Tbsp Gabriel friendly cooking oil (see page 24)
500g marinated roo steaks

Method:
Roo steaks can be purchased marinated and we find this is the best way to buy them to ensure their tenderness.
1. If using home-made marinade, remove steaks from fridge 30 minutes prior to cooking.
2. If steaks are thick, slice them lengthways to assist with cooking.
3. Melt cooking oil onto frying pan or BBQ on medium-high heat.
4. Place steaks on hot BBQ or frying pan. Cook on each side for approximately 2 minutes or until cooked to your liking. Be careful not to overcook as meat will become tough. We prefer our roo steaks cooked medium-rare.
5. Serve with salad.

Home-Made Marinade

Preparation time: 10 minutes
Marinating time: minimum 4 hours, though overnight is recommended

Ingredients:
¼ cup balsamic vinegar
½ cup Gabriel friendly cooking oil
1 Tbsp fresh rosemary, finely chopped
1 Tbsp thyme, fresh or dried
2 cloves garlic, crushed
½ tsp pepper to taste

Method:
1. Combine all ingredients together in marinating dish.
2. If roo steaks are thick, cut them lengthways to assist with cooking.
3. Place steaks in dish and cover with marinade. Refrigerate for a minimum of 4 hours.

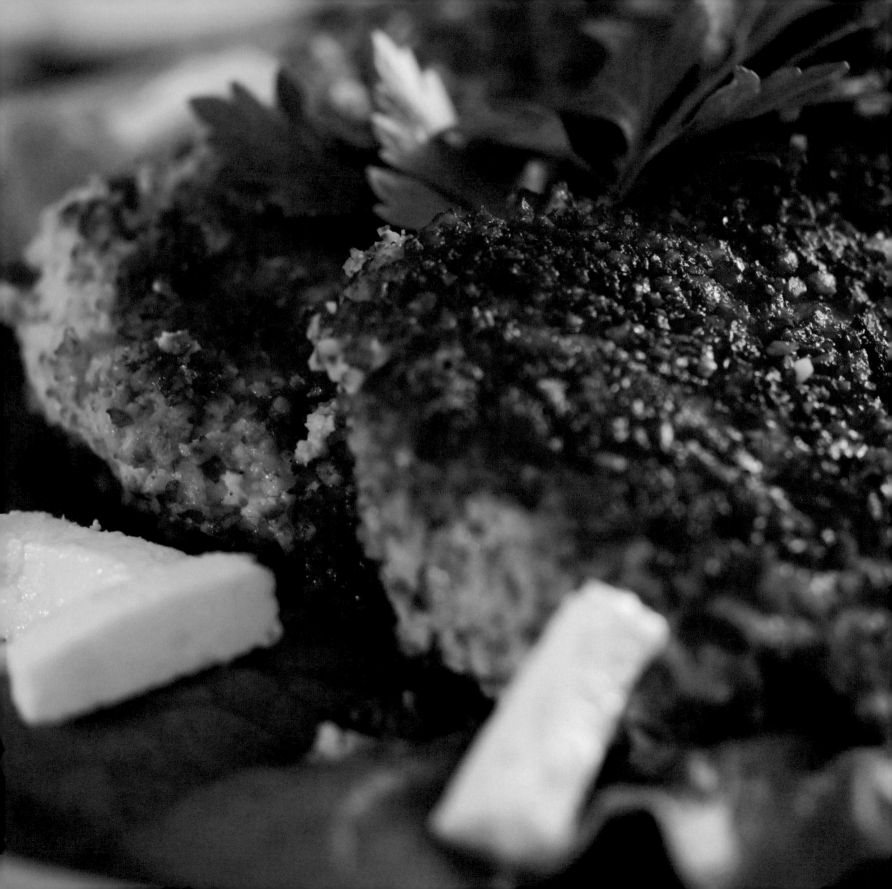

"Crispy and crunchy without the bread crumbs."

Almond Chicken

Serves: 4
Preparation time: 15 minutes
Cooking time: 10 minutes

Ingredients:
4 chicken thigh fillets (organic, free range)
1 egg yolk, beaten
1 cup ground almonds
pinch healthy salt (see page 17)
parsley to serve
Gabriel friendly cooking oil (see page 24)

Method:
1. Place egg yolk in one bowl and ground almonds and salt in another bowl.
2. Dip each chicken fillet into egg yolk, be sure to cover both sides. Dip chicken into almonds so that both sides are coated.
3. Heat cooking oil in frying pan on medium to high heat. Cook chicken for approximately 4-5 minutes on each side or until cooked through.
4. Serve with a fresh salad.

Pork Fillet with Caramelised Apple

Serves: 2
Preparation time: 10 minutes
Cooking time: 15 minutes

Ingredients:
350g pork fillet, cut into 1cm rounds
1 apple, peeled and cubed
1 Tbsp Gabriel friendly cooking oil (see page 24)
¼ tsp xylitol
¼ tsp cinnamon
¼ tsp cumin

Method:
1. Heat cooking oil in frying pan on medium heat. Add apples to pan with xylitol and cook for 2-3 minutes stirring from time to time. Add the cumin and cinnamon and stir through. Reduce heat, cover and cook until apples are tender. Adding 1 tablespoon of water will create a steaming effect to tenderise apples. Remove from pan and set aside.
2. Increase heat and add more oil to pan if required. Place pork slices in pan and cook for a few minutes on each side until cooked to your liking. Return apple to pan and cook for another minute. Season with salt and pepper before serving.

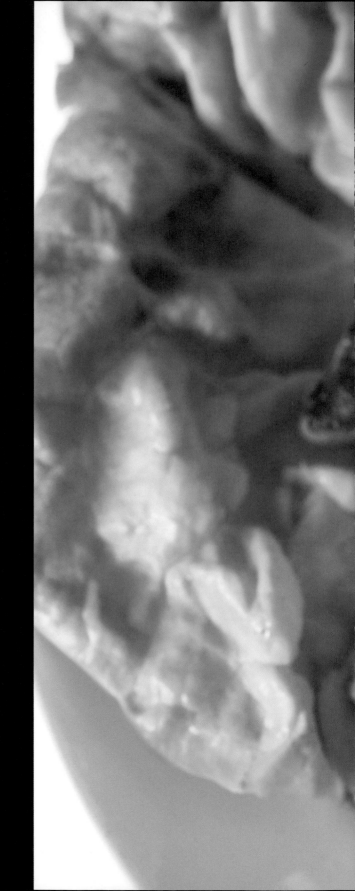

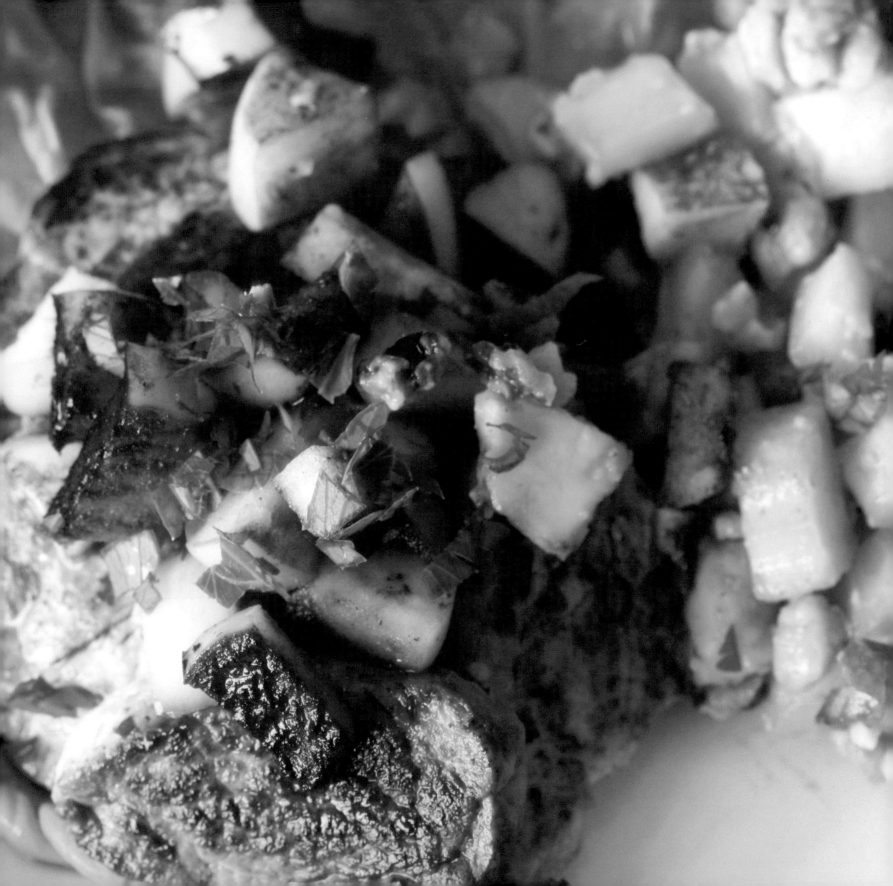

Spicy Meatballs with Asian Greens

Serves: 4
Preparation time: 15 minutes
Cooking time: 20 minutes

Ingredients:

2 Tbsp Gabriel friendly cooking oil (see page 24)
1 brown onion, finely chopped
2 tsp ginger, finely grated
1 tsp chinese five spice*
*A combination of cinnamon, star anise, fennel, cloves and pepper

600g beef (organic grass-fed) mince
40ml plum sauce
1 Tbsp tamari
4 bok choy

Method:

1. Heat 1 Tbsp cooking oil in frying pan over medium heat. Add onion and cook for approximately 3 minutes or until softened. Add ginger and Chinese Five Spice. Cook, stirring for 1 minute. Set aside to cool for approximately 5 minutes.
2. Transfer onion mixture to large mixing bowl. Add mince meat and mix with hands to combine.
3. Roll mince mixture into meatballs, using approximately 1 Tbsp of mixture for each meatball.
4. In cleaned frying pan melt 1 Tbsp cooking oil on medium-high heat. Add the meatballs and cook for 6-8 minutes, turning from time to time to ensure they are cooked through.
5. Add plum sauce and tamari and stir until meatballs are well coated.
6. Place bok choy in pan over meatballs. Cover and cook for another 1-2 minutes to lightly steam the bok choy.

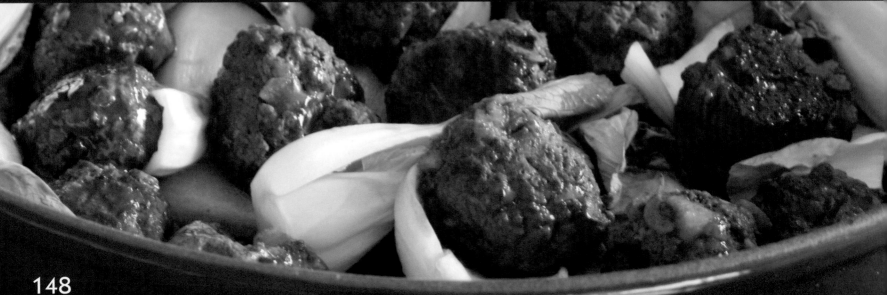

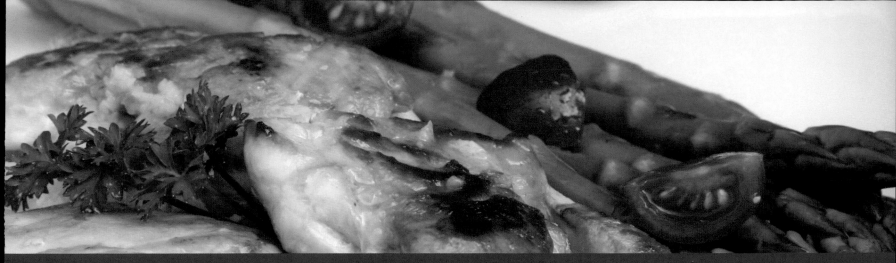

Chicken and Asparagus with Lemon Butter Sauce

Serves: 2
Preparation time: 10 minutes
Cooking time: 15 minutes

Ingredients:

1 Tbsp Gabriel friendly cooking oil (see page 24)
4 chicken thigh fillets
1 Tbsp tamari
1 bunch asparagus (approximately 12 spears)

25g butter
juice of half a lemon
2 cloves garlic crushed
1 Tbsp flax seeds

Method:

For the chicken:
Cut chicken fillets in half length ways. Heat cooking oil in frying pan on medium-high heat. Place chicken in pan. Cook for approximately 3-4 minutes. Add tamari. Turn chicken fillets over and cook for another 3-4 minutes or until chicken is cooked through.

For the asparagus:
Cut approximately 3 cm off ends of asparagus. Steam asparagus for approximately 2-3 minutes. You only want the colour to darken slightly.

For the lemon butter sauce:
Place butter, lemon juice and crushed garlic in small pan on low-medium heat. Once butter has melted, remove from heat.

To serve: Place chicken and asparagus on plate. Serve with salad. Drizzle with 1-2 tablespoons of sauce and sprinkle with flax seeds.

Tandoori Fish Curry

Serves: 4
Preparation time: 10 minutes
Cooking time: 10 minutes

Ingredients:
2 Tbsp tandoori paste
⅔ cup coconut milk
2 cloves garlic, crushed
600g fish, firm white flesh, cut into strips
1 Tbsp Gabriel friendly cooking oil (see page 24)
fresh parsley, to serve
lemon wedges, to serve

Method:
1. Place tandoori paste, coconut milk and garlic in a medium bowl. Whisk together to combine.
2. Add fish to bowl and stir through to cover all fish pieces in sauce.
3. Heat cooking oil in frying pan on medium to high heat.
4. Add fish and sauce to pan. Cook, stirring, for 5 minutes.
5. Serve with fresh parsley and lemon wedges.

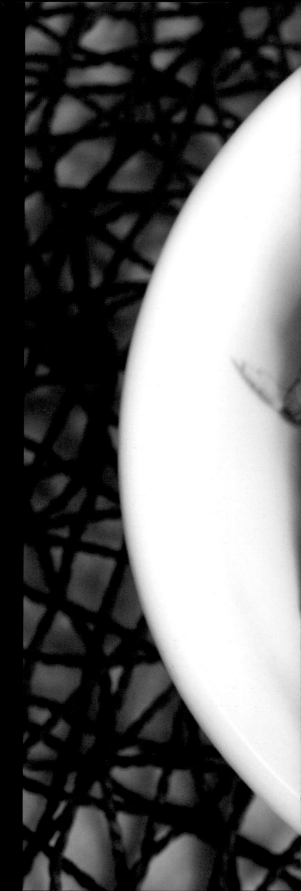

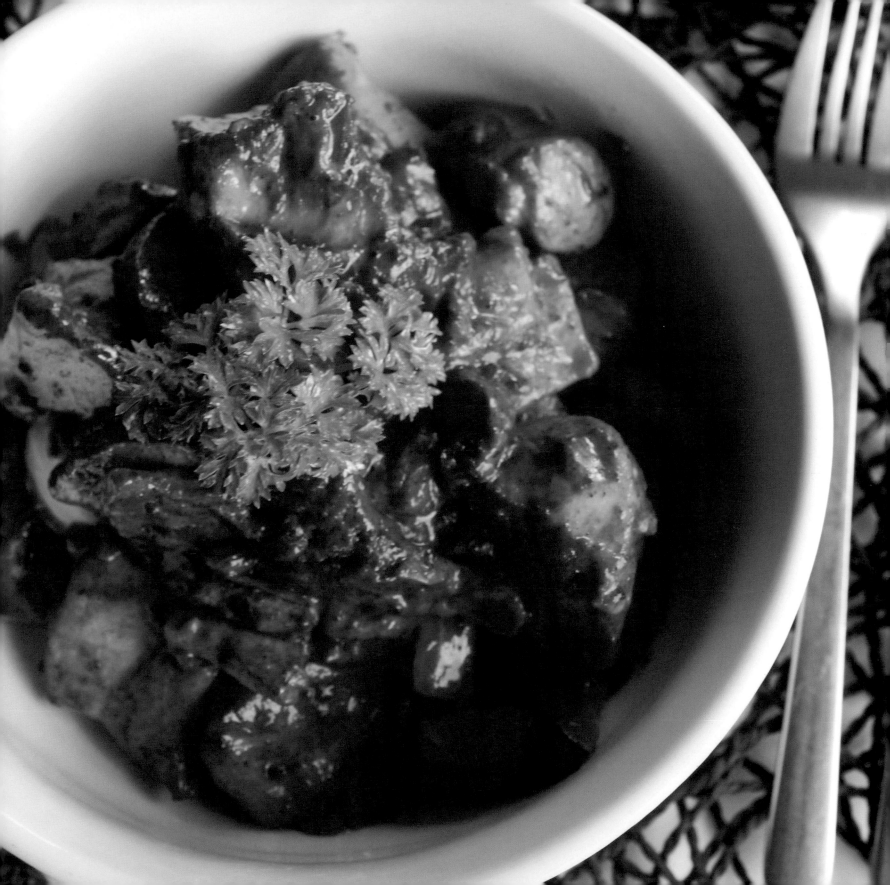

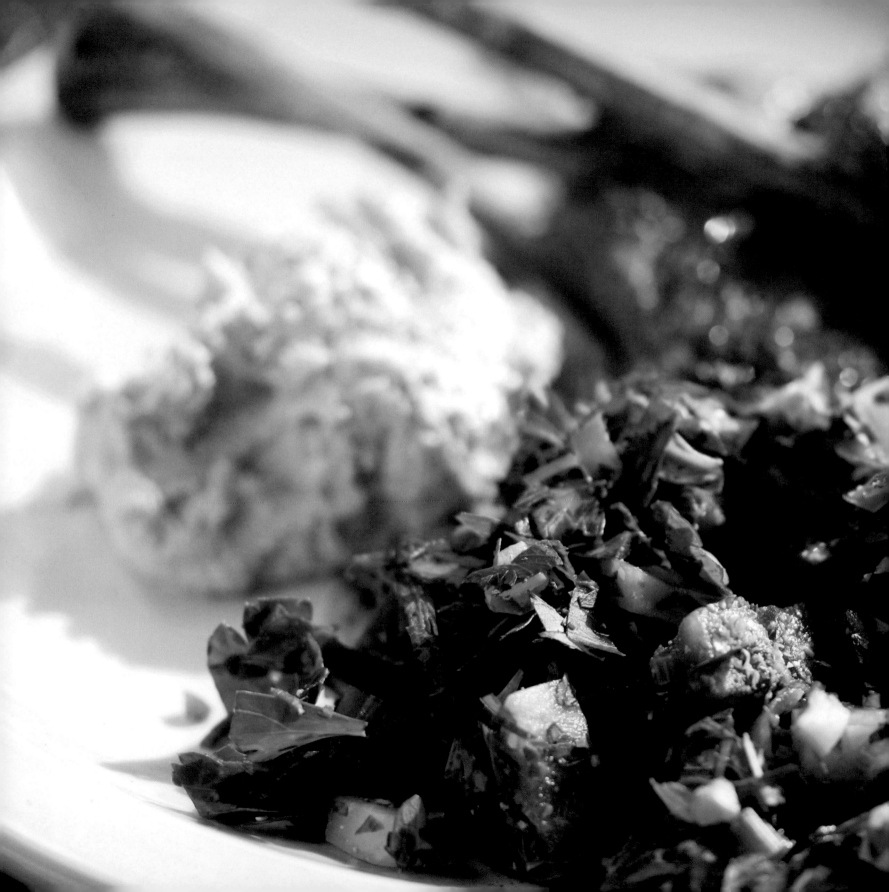

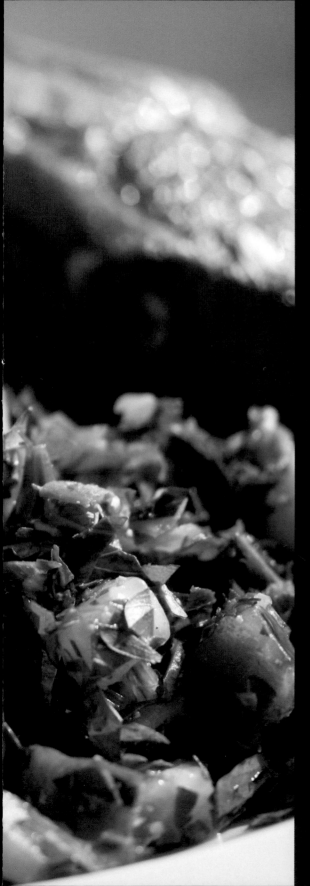

Rosemary Lamb Cutlets

Serves: 4
Preparation time: 10 minutes
Cooking time: 10 minutes

Ingredients:
12 lamb cutlets
1 Tbsp Gabriel friendly cooking oil (see page 24)
2 Tbsp rosemary, finely chopped
healthy salt (see page 17) and pepper

Method:
1. Combine rosemary, oil, salt and pepper in medium bowl.
   Roll lamb cutlets in rosemary mixture.
2. Heat cooking oil in frying pan or on BBQ on medium-high heat. Cook lamb cutlets for 2-3 minutes on each side or until cooked to your liking.
3. Perfectly accompanied by Tabouli (see page 188) and Hummus (see page 63).

"An incredibly easy, deliciously tasty and happily healthy meal!"

Seared Salmon

Serves: 4
Preparation time: 5 minutes
Cooking time: 5 minutes

Ingredients:
4 salmon steaks (approximately 600g)

Method:
1. Place frying pan on stove top on high heat.
2. Once the pan is very hot, wash the salmon in water. Do not dry it. Place it directly on the hot pan. Cook for 2 minutes before flipping over to cook the other side.
3. Serve immediately with fresh crunchy greens.

Baked Salmon Pesto

Serves: 4
Preparation time: 20 minutes
Cooking time: 25 minutes

Ingredients:

4 salmon fillets (600g)

4 Tbsp pesto

2 spring onions (scallions), sliced

100g cherry tomatoes, quartered

200ml dry white wine

150ml fish stock (with no MSG, artificial colours or flavours)

salt and pepper

Method:

1. Preheat oven to 180°C / 355°F
2. Place the 4 salmon fillets into a deep baking dish. Spread 1 Tbsp of pesto over each fillet and cover with tomatoes and spring onions (scallions).
3. In a medium saucepan, combine wine and stock. Boil and season with salt and pepper. Pour liquid over salmon.
4. Place baking dish in oven and cook for approximately 25 minutes or until salmon breaks easily away from itself when cut.

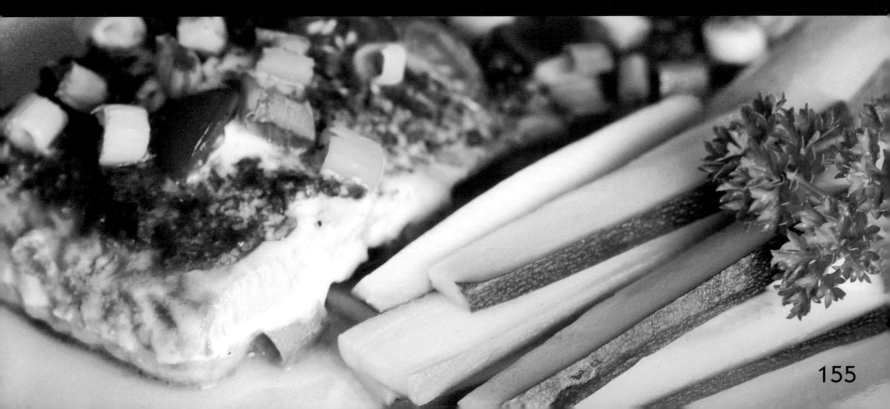

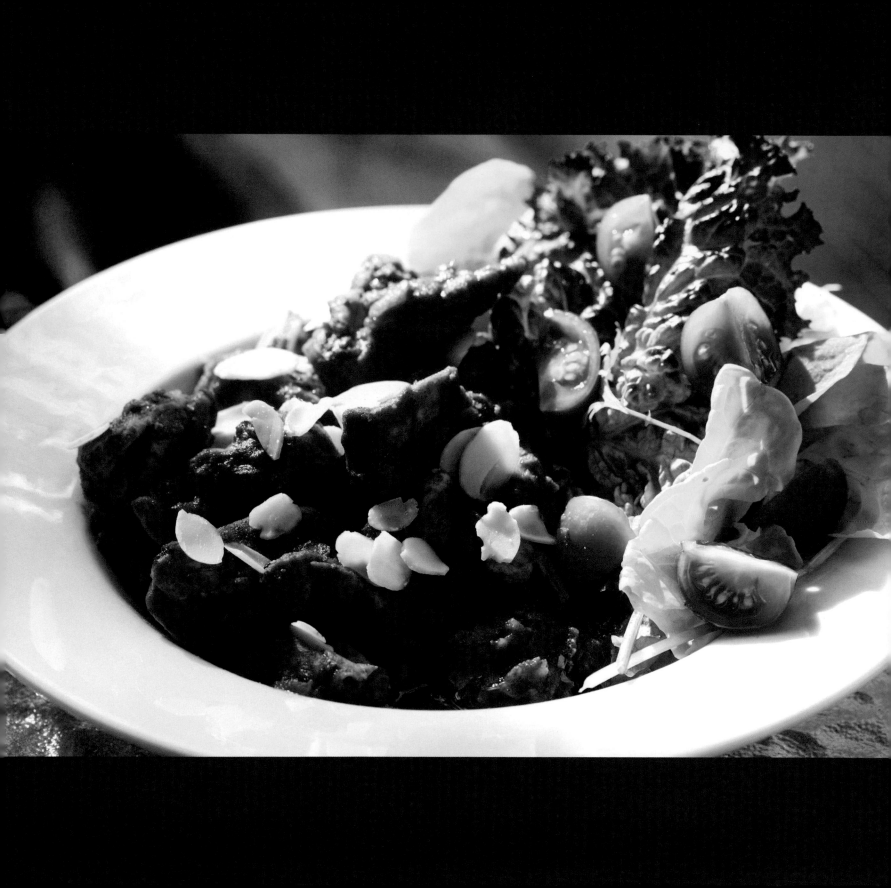

Butter Chicken

Serves: 4
Preparation time: 30 minutes
Cooking time: 20 minutes

Ingredients:

2 onions, diced finely
3 garlic cloves, peeled and crushed
4cm fresh ginger, grated
1 red chilli (optional), sliced thinly
4 chicken thigh fillets (organic, free range),
cut into thick strips
1 Tbsp Gabriel friendly cooking oil (see page 24)
25g butter
1 Tbsp cumin seeds, crushed
1 Tbsp fennel seeds, crushed
4 cardamom pods

1 Tbsp ground paprika
1 Tbsp ground turmeric
1 tsp ground cinnamon
300ml chicken stock (with no MSG, artificial colours
or flavours)
2 Tbsp tomato puree
¼ cup natural yoghurt
pinch of salt
2 Tbsp flaked almonds, to serve coriander sprigs,
to serve

Method:

1. Combine onions, garlic, ginger and chilli.
2. Heat cooking oil in a frying pan and cook chicken in batches, turning each piece until all chicken is browned on both sides. Remove chicken from pan and set aside on absorbant paper.
3. Add butter to the pan. Once it has melted add the onion mix. Cook while stirring for 1 minute. Add to pan cumin, fennel, cardamom, paprika, turmeric, cinnamon. Cook for another minute before adding stock, tomato puree and salt. Stir continuously until mixture begins to boil.
4. Return chicken to pan. Spoon mixture over chicken. Cover and cook on low-medium heat for 10 minutes. Add yoghurt and stir it through. Garnish with flaked almonds and coriander prior to serving.

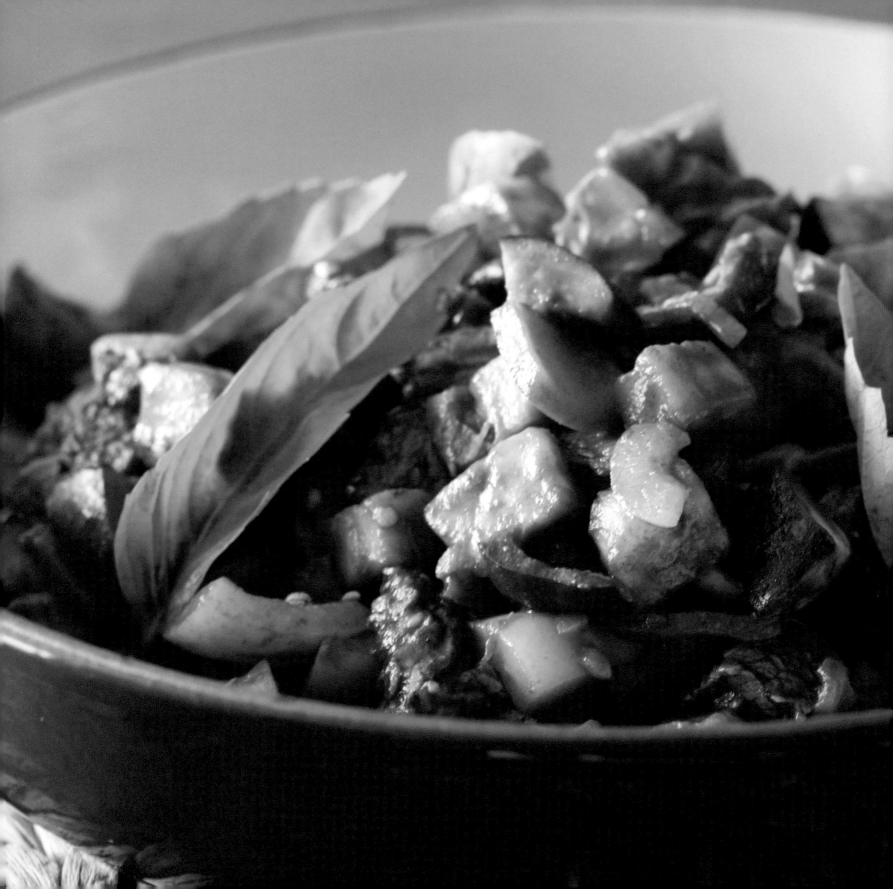

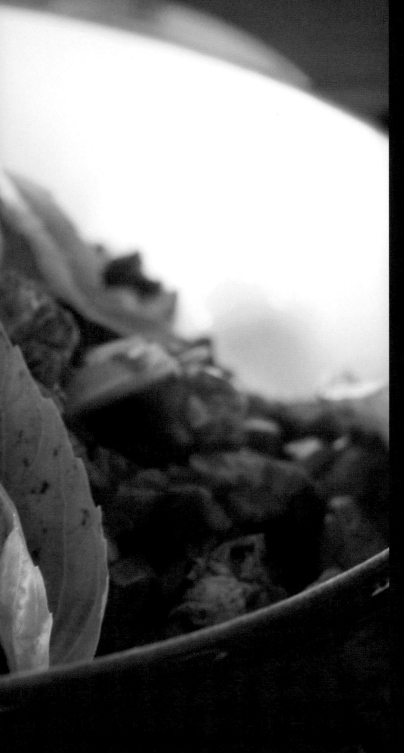

Beefed Up Ratatouille

Serves: 4
Preparation time: 15 minutes
Cooking time: 15 minutes

Ingredients:
2 Tbsp Gabriel Method-friendly cooking oil
500g beef (organic grass-fed) braising steak,cubed
8 tomatoes, cubed or 2 tins organic tomatoes
1 large onion, chopped finely
1 red capsicum (bell pepper), cut lengthways into strips
1 yellow capsicum (bell pepper), cut lengthways into strips
½ green capsicum (bell pepper), cut lengthways into strips
1 eggplant, cubed
1 Tbsp tomato paste
½ Tbsp fresh thyme leaves
2 Tbsp fresh basil, chopped
2 garlic cloves, peeled and crushed
1 beef stock cube (with no MSG, artificial colours or flavours)

Method:
1. Heat oil in pan on medium to high heat. Add beef to pan in batches, cooking until lightly browned on all sides though do not cook through. Remove and set aside.
2. Cook onions and garlic on medium heat. Return beef to pan. Add capsicum (bell pepper) and eggplant pieces and tomato paste. Cook for 5 minutes, stirring.
3. Add chopped tomatoes, stock cube, basil and thyme. Stir through until stock cube has entirely dissolved. Season with salt and pepper. Cook for a further 5 minutes. Serve hot.

Pizza-Topped Chicken

Serves: 4
Preparation time: 15 minutes
Cooking time: 15 minutes

Ingredients:
2 (approximately 650g) organic free range chicken breast fillets
1 Tbsp Gabriel friendly cooking oil (see page 24)
4 tsp pizza sauce
12 baby spinach leaves
1 mushroom, sliced very thinly
½ small onion, sliced very thinly
¼ cup cheddar cheese, grated
¼ cup mozzarella cheese, grated

Method:
1. Cut chicken fillets in half lengthways.
2. Heat cooking oil in frying pan on medium to high heat. Cook chicken on both sides for approximately 3 minutes or until just cooked through. To assist with cooking, place a lid on the frying pan and reduce heat to low. Cook for 2 minutes or until cooked through.
3. Remove chicken from pan and place onto a flat surface. Heat grill to medium to high heat.
4. Top each half fillet with 1 tsp tomato paste, 3 baby spinach leaves, mushrooms and onions. Transfer chicken fillets to the grill, distribute the cheese over the 4 fillets. Grill for 2 minutes or until cheese has melted and turned golden.
5. Serve with salad.

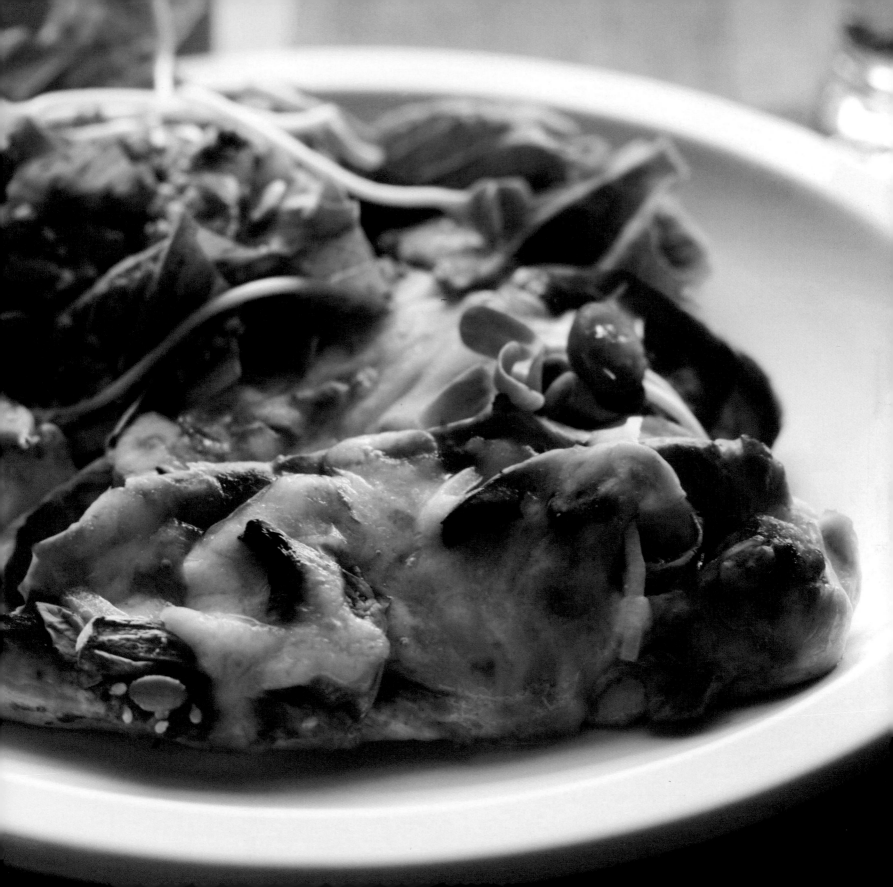

Roo Burger with Chilli Tahini Sauce

Serves: 4
Preparation time: 20 minutes + 30 minutes refrigeration time
Cooking time: 5 minutes

Ingredients:
400g roo mince (or other organic grassfed mince)
2 spring onions (scallions), chopped finely
1 clove garlic, peeled and crushed
1 egg yolk
1 tsp dried sage
1 tsp fresh or dried thyme
salt and pepper
Gabriel friendly cooking oil (see page 24)

Method:
1. Place all ingredients for the roo burgers in a bowl. Mix together until all ingredients are well combined.
2. Divide the mixture up into 4 equal parts. Shape each part into a ball and refrigerate for 30 minutes.
3. To cook your burgers, heat cooking oil in frying pan on medium heat. Once the oil is hot place roo patties into pan. Press down on them with an egg flip to flatten. Cook on each side for 2-3 minutes or until cooked to your liking.
4. Serve on a bed of lettuce with salad ingredients and Chilli Tahini Sauce (see page 204)

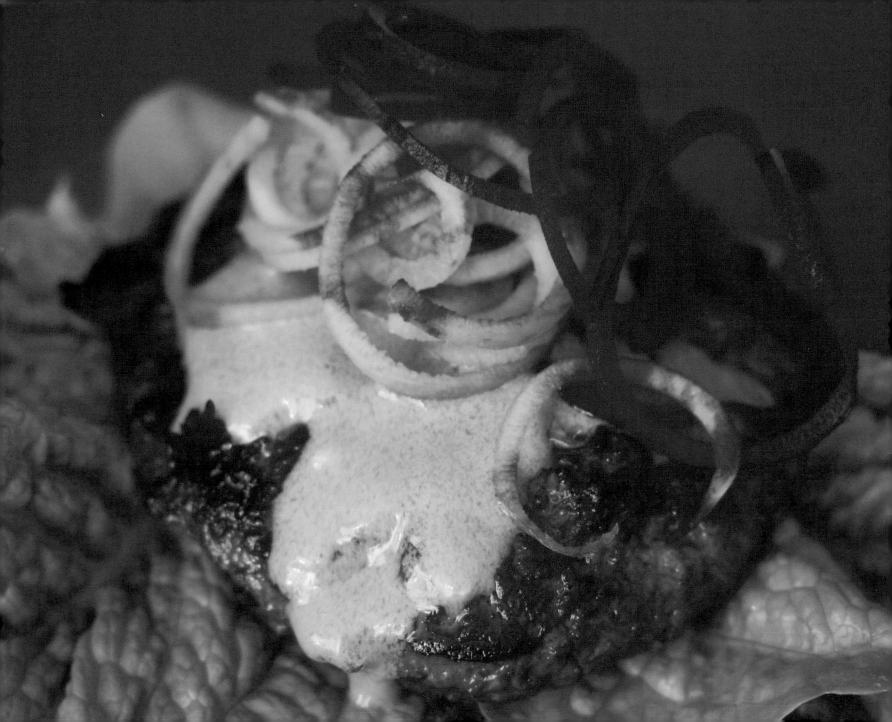

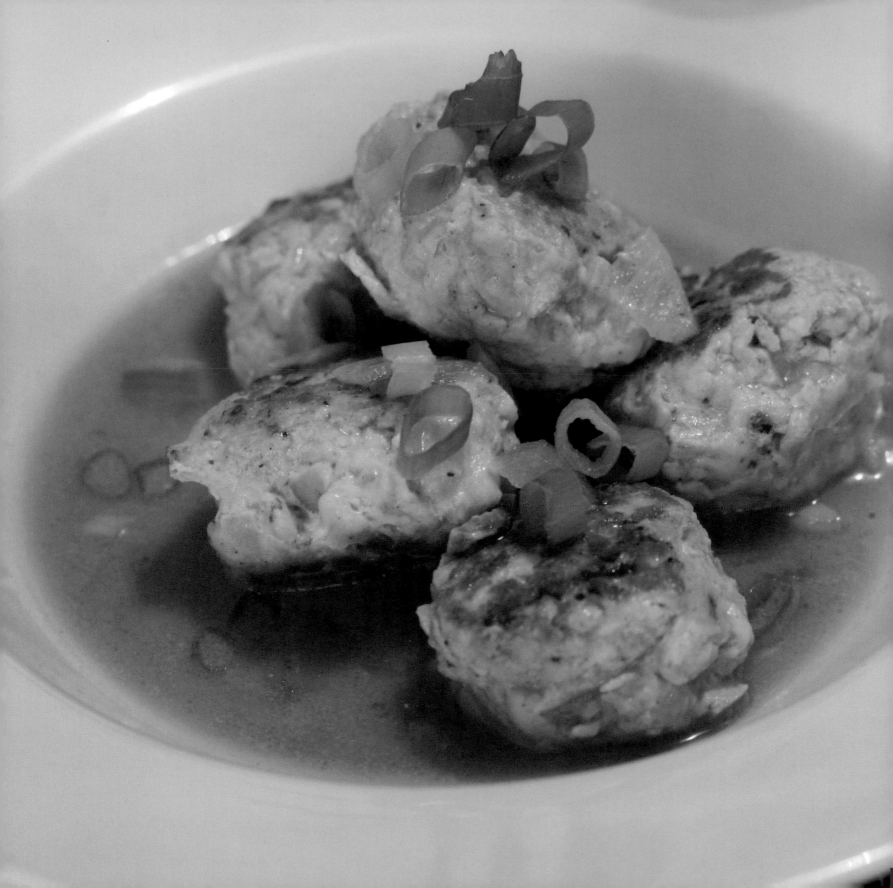

Turkey Meatballs

Serves: 4
Preparation time: 20 minutes
Cooking time: 20 minutes

Note: Minced (ground) chicken or pork can also be used with this recipe

Ingredients:
For the meatballs:
1 onion, diced finely
500g minced (ground) turkey (organic, free range)
1 egg yolk
1-2 Tbsp Gabriel friendly cooking oil (see page 24)
healthy salt (see page 17) and pepper

For the Sauce:
50g butter
1 onion, sliced
250ml chicken stock (with no MSG, artificial colours or flavours)
3 tsp Dijon mustard
½ tsp turmeric

Method:
To make the meatballs:
1. In a bowl, mix together onion, turkey, egg yolk, salt and pepper. Shape the mixture into 20 small meatballs.
2. Heat cooking oil in a large frying pan on high heat. Cook meatballs in batches, turning them while cooking until they are evenly browned all over. Remove from pan and place onto a plate with absorbent paper. Wipe the pan clean with paper towel between batches and reapply oil if necessary.

To make the Sauce:
1. Melt the butter in a frying pan on low-medium heat. Add onion and fry approximately 5 minutes or until softened. Gradually stir in the stock and boil. Add mustard, turmeric, salt and pepper and stir until combined.
2. Place meatballs into the sauce. Spoon the sauce over meatballs so that they are covered. Cook on low-medium heat for approximately 15 minutes or until meatballs are cooked through.

Satay Chicken Stir Fry

Serves: 4
Preparation time: 15 minutes
Cooking time: 20 minutes

Ingredients for the Satay Sauce:
1 Tbsp Gabriel friendly cooking oil (see page 24)
2 cloves garlic, crushed
3cm piece of ginger
½ fresh red chilli, seeds removed, sliced thinly
2 Tbsp organic peanut butter, sugar free
1 Tbsp tamari
1 Tbsp coconut palm sugar
1 Tbsp lime juice
salt to season

Ingredients for the Stir Fry:
600g chicken breast fillet, thinly sliced
1 red capsicum (bell pepper), thinly sliced
1 cup bean sprouts
150g snow peas
3 bok choy
1 garlic clove, crushed
pinch pepper
fresh coriander
shallots
lime wedges

Method:
1. For the sauce: In a medium saucepan, heat cooking oil over medium heat. Fry garlic, ginger and chilli until tender. Add peanut butter and allow to melt then add tamari, coconut palm sugar, lime juice and salt to taste. Remove from heat and cover.
2. Heat a wok or large frying pan over medium to high heat. Cook the chicken in batches stir frying each batch for 2-3 minutes or until golden brown. Add extra cooking oil between batches if necessary.
   Using a slotted spoon, transfer all the chicken to a plate and set aside.
3. Add capsicum (bell pepper), bean sprouts, snow peas, bok choy and garlic. Stir fry until vegetables become tender. Return chicken to the pan and add pepper.
4. Divide stir fry into 4 bowls. Drizzle with the satay sauce and garnish with coriander, shallots and a lime wedge.

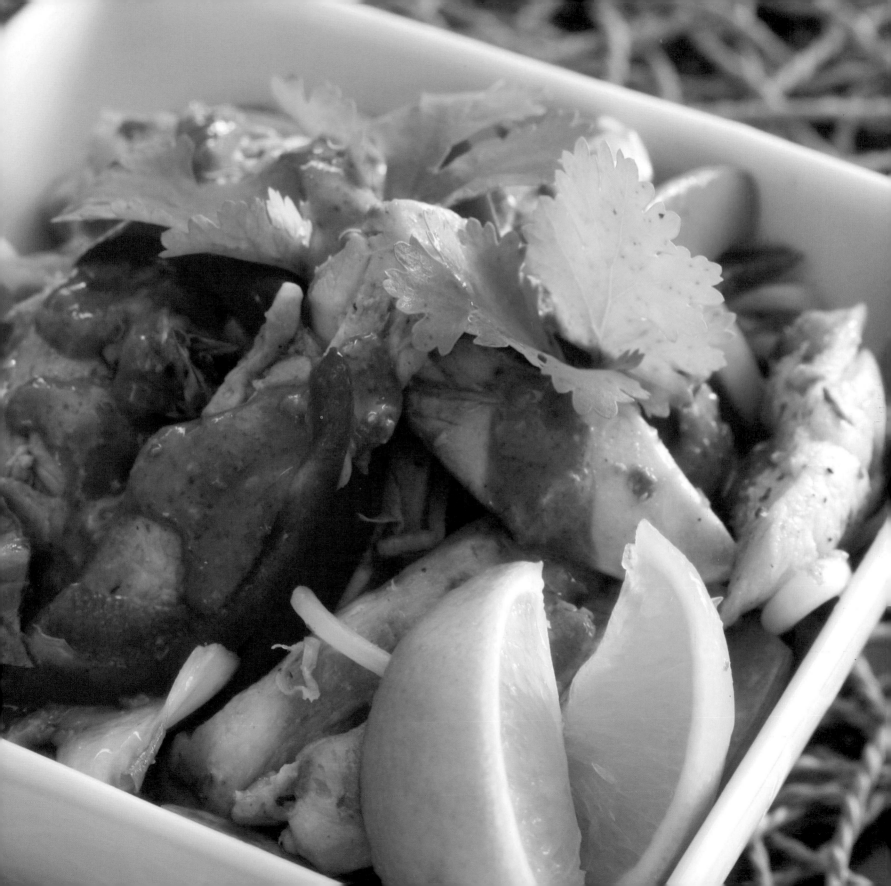

Beef & Grilled Vegetable Moussaka

Serves: 6
Preparation time: 60 minutes
Cooking time: 80 minutes

Ingredients for the Meat Sauce:
1 Tbsp Gabriel Method-friendly cooking oil
1 onion, chopped finely
500g organic grass fed minced (ground) beef
6 fresh tomatoes, diced or 2 tins organic tomatoes
1 tsp oregano, fresh or dried
2 cloves garlic, peeled and crushed

Ingredients for the Topping:
½ cup cheddar cheese, grated
½ cup mozzarella cheese, grated
¼ cup Parmesan cheese, grated

Ingredients for the Roast Vegetables:
1 red capsicum (bell pepper), deseeded and cut lengthways into strips
1 yellow capsicum (bell pepper), deseeded and cut lengthways into strips
2 medium eggplants, cut lengthways into ½ cm slices
3 zucchini, cut lengthways into ½ cm slices
Gabriel friendly cooking oil (see page 24)

Method:
1. For the meat sauce, heat cooking oil in frying pan on low– medium heat. Add onion to pan and cook until onion begins to soften (approximately 3 minutes).
2. Increase heat to medium. Add mince and cook, stirring, for 3 to 4 minutes or until meat begins to brown. Add tomato, oregano and garlic. Allow to boil then reduce heat, cover and simmer for 10-15 minutes or until sauce begins to thicken.
3. Preheat grill to a medium heat. In batches, place capsicum (bell pepper), eggplant and zucchini onto grill tray. Brush with oil. Cook on each side for approximately 6 minutes or until it begins to darken in colour. Transfer vegetables to a plate and set aside.

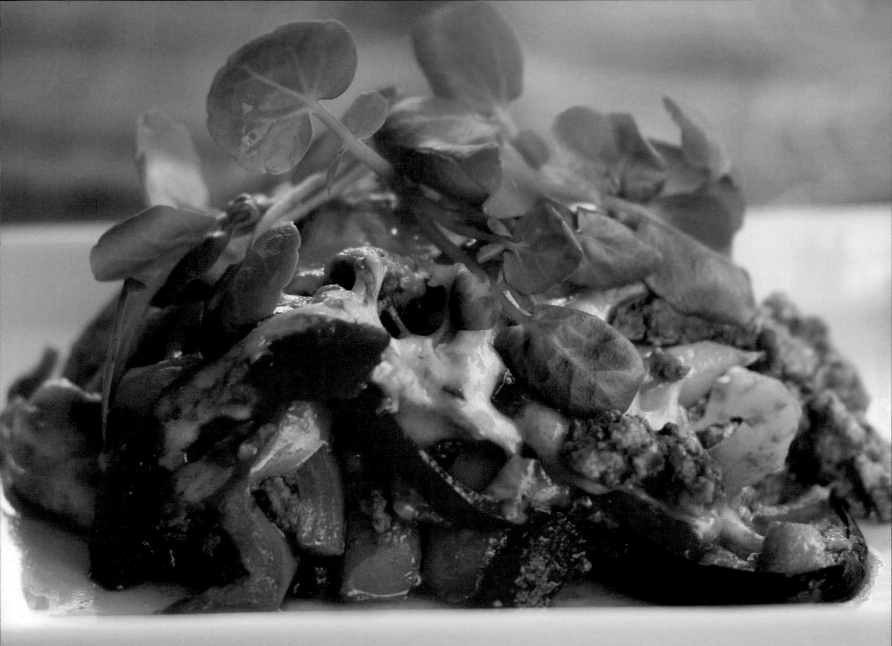

4. Preheat oven to 180°C / 355°F. In a large baking dish, layer vegetables and meat sauce with eggplant at the base followed by zucchini and half the meat sauce. Add another layer of eggplant followed by capsicum (bell pepper) and the remaining meat sauce. Top with the three cheeses.
5. Place moussaka in the oven and cook for 35-40 minutes.
6. Allow to cool for 5 minutes prior to serving. Serve with a tasty green salad.

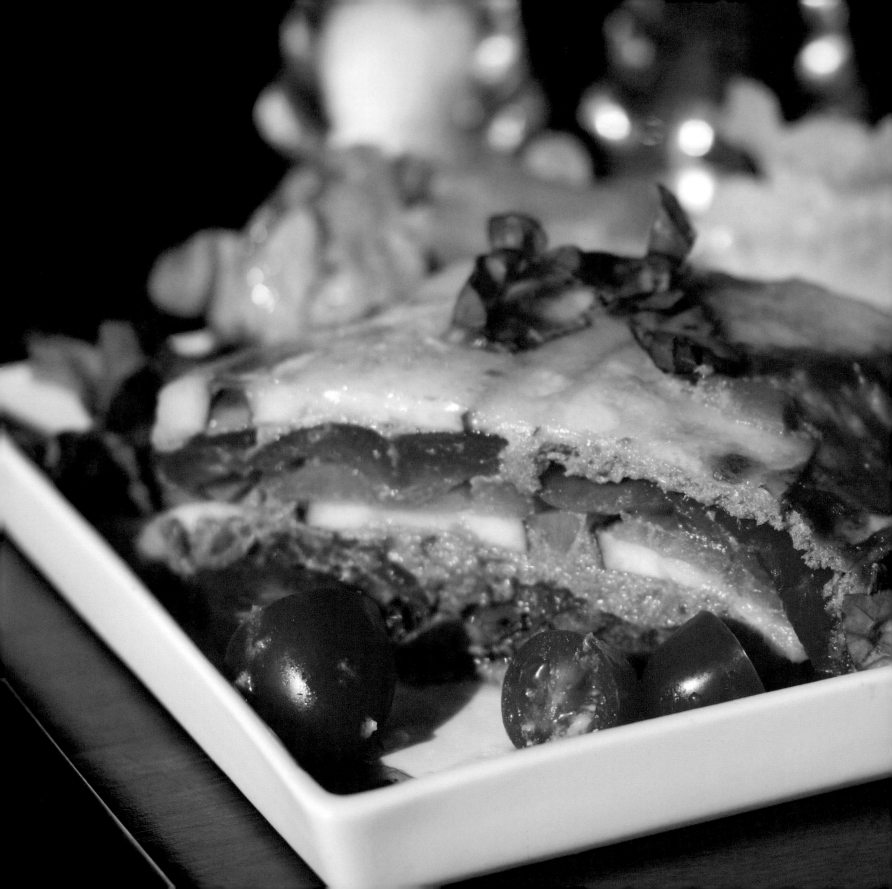

"An interesting variation on the traditional lasagne. Here we use zucchini instead of pasta with a salmon based sauce, full of Omega-3s."

Zucchini and Salmon Lasagne

Serves: 4-6
Preparation time: 60 minutes
Cooking time: 30 minutes

Ingredients:
2 cups silverbeet, steamed
2 cups carrot, sliced thinly, lengthways, steamed
1 cup red onion, sliced, steamed
1 cup roasted capsicum (bell pepper), sliced lengthways
2 medium zucchini, sliced thinly, lengthways
1 cup mozzarella, grated
¼ cup Parmesan, shaved or grated

For the Sauce:
400g salmon
150g tomato paste
¼ cup lemon juice
1 cup ricotta
½ cup fresh basil
½ cup fresh oregano

Method:
1. Preheat oven to 180°C / 355°F. Grease 2 litre capacity baking dish.
2. Make the sauce by placing all sauce ingredients in food processor, mix until well combined.
3. At the base of the baking dish, place all the silverbeet and half the carrots, half the onions and half the capsicum (bell pepper). Cover with half the sauce.
4. Now layer half the zucchini plus the remaining carrot, onion and capsicum (bell pepper). Cover with remaining sauce.
5. Place the rest of the zucchini on top. Sprinkle with mozzarella and Parmesan.
6. Bake in oven for 30-40 minutes or until browned.
7. Serve with scrumptious salad.

Roast Turkey with Gabriel Method 'Stuffing' and Greens

Serves: 8
Preparation time: 15 minutes
Cooking time: 3 hours

Ingredients:
4 ½ kg turkey (preferably organic
free range)
Gabriel friendly cooking oil
(see page 24)
2 sprigs fresh thyme
1 sprig fresh rosemary
salt and pepper to season
1 cup water

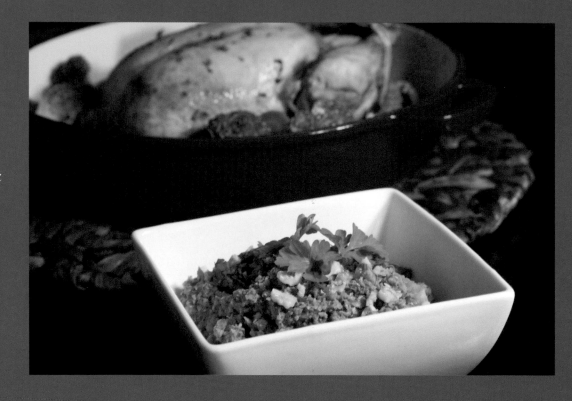

Method:
1. Preheat oven to 180°C / 355°F.
2. Rinse the inside and outside of the turkey under cold water. Pat dry with paper towel. Place turkey, breast side down, in a baking dish.
3. If stuffing the turkey, spoon the mixture into the cavity. Tie the legs together with kitchen string. Brush cooking oil over the turkey and sprinkle with thyme and rosemary leaves, salt and pepper. Pour one cup of water into the base of the baking dish.
4. Reduce oven temperature to 160°C / 320°F. Place turkey in oven and roast for 1 hour. Remove from oven, baste it with juices in pan and turn it over so that it is now breast side up. Baste every 30 minutes, for another 1½ to 2 hours or until juices run clear when thigh is pierced with a skewer. A stuffed turkey will require more cooking time.
5. When turkey is cooked, remove from oven and cover with foil. Set aside to rest for 10-15 minutes.

Gabriel Method 'Stuffing'

Use this tasty stuffing for your roast chickens and festive turkeys. Either cook it as an accompaniment (by following the recipe) or simply fill your chicken or turkey with the uncooked, chopped up ingredients prior to roasting.

Serves: 8
Preparation time: 15 minutes
Cooking time: 30 minutes

Ingredients:
2 Tbsp Gabriel friendly cooking oil (see page 24)
2 red onions, diced
4 spring onions (scallions), cut finely
1 fennel bulb, cut into long thin strips
2 stalks celery, cubed
1 cup chicken stock (with no MSG, artificial colours or flavours)
2 large mushrooms, sliced thinly
½ cup walnuts, chopped (or pan roasted if you prefer a more crunchy consistency)
½ tsp sage
2 cloves garlic, crushed
¼ cup red wine (optional)
salt and pepper to taste
1 Tbsp fresh parsley, to serve

Method:
1. Heat oil in frying pan on medium heat. Add onions, spring onions, fennel and celery. Stir for several minutes to coat vegetables in oil until lightly browned.
2. Add chicken stock, stir through and increase heat to Boil. Reduce heat to low and cover pan. Simmer for 5 minutes.
3. Add mushrooms, walnuts, sage, garlic and wine. Season as required with salt and pepper. Stir through and allow to simmer on low heat for another 10 minutes.
4. Serve warm, sprinkled with fresh parsley. Or refrigerate and reheat when ready to serve.

Greens with Almond and Lemon

Serves: 8
Preparation time: 10 minutes
Cooking time: 10 minutes

Ingredients:
2 tsp Gabriel friendly cooking oil (see page 24)
1 tsp lemon rind, grated
1 Tbsp lemon juice
2 bunches broccolini
2 bunches asparagus
150g sugar snap peas
¼ cup flaked almonds

Method:
1. Place cooking oil, lemon rind and lemon juice in a glass jar. Tighten lid and shake to combine.
2. Lightly toast almonds in a dry frying pan over medium heat.
3. Lightly steam broccolini, asparagus, sugar snap peas for 1 minute or until they are bright green in colour. Place steamed greens in serving dish. Top with almonds and drizzle with lemon mixture to serve.

"A great tasting side dish for any meat or fish recipe."

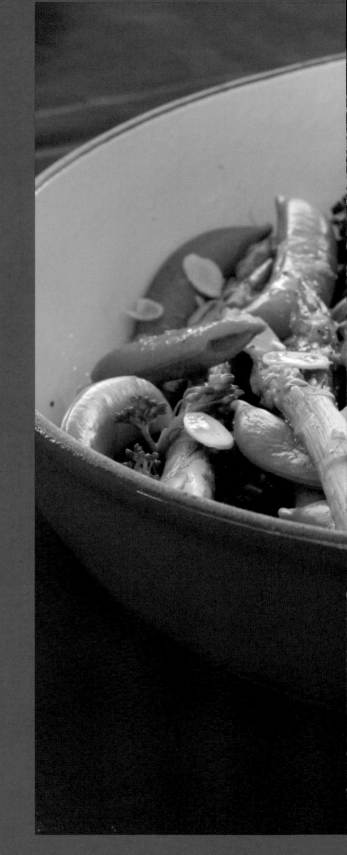

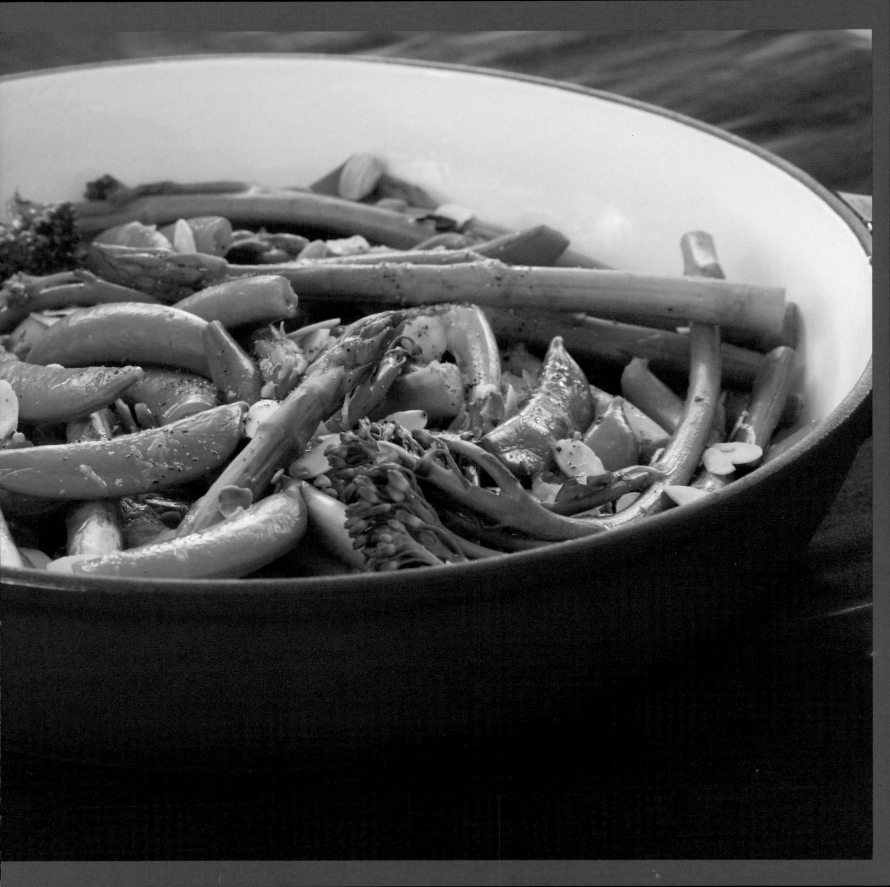

Life-Force Foods

This part of the book features nutrient rich, high vitality live foods. Salads are a big focus here, for obvious reasons, but we're also including fresh-extracted vegetable juices.

Living foods are essential eating. Live foods are rich in enzymes that help with digestion and are also full of easily assimilable proteins, vitamins, minerals, essential oils and carbohydrates. The high alkalinity and water content of live foods also helps to eliminate toxins and cellular waste products.

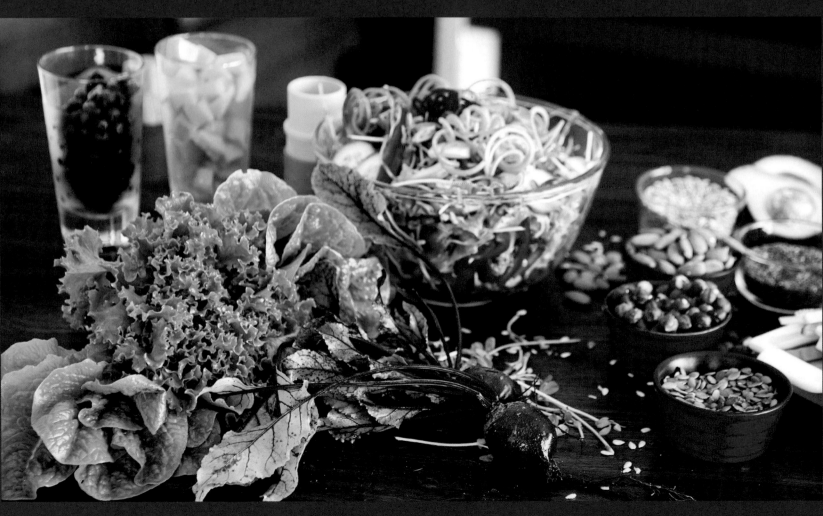

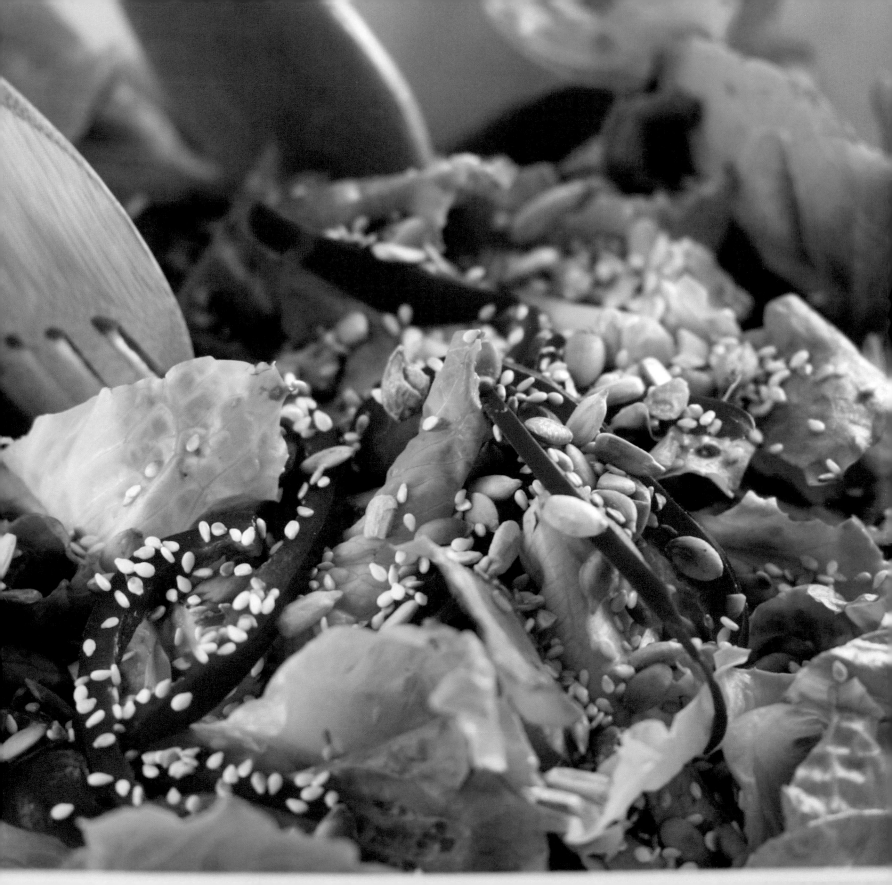

Life-Force Foods

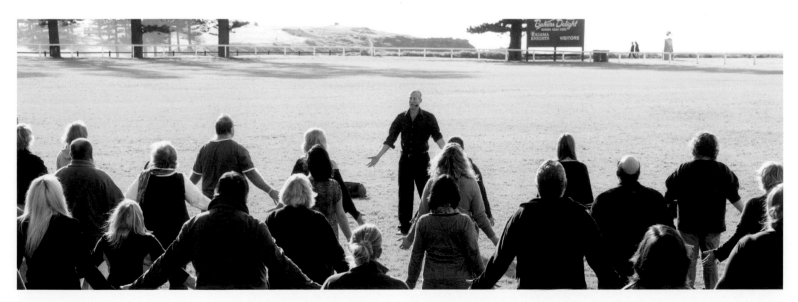

Make It a Salad

Absolutely any meal can be made into a salad.

We recommend doing so for several reasons:

- You're getting all the advantages of live foods.
- You're eating more slowly
- You're consuming more high water content food so you are hydrating your body
- You are also nourishing and detoxifying your body

If you use a healthy salad dressing with lots of flaxseed, linseed or chia – either ground or in the form of cold-pressed oil – it's a great way to get your Omega-3s. You'll begin to develop a real taste for salad and begin to crave it, rather than craving dead carbs.

Research suggests that overeating cooked foods can trigger a toxic immune response in your body called leukocytosis, which results in elevation of white blood cells and overstimulation of the immune response, which in turn results in inflammation and stress - a chronic trigger for the FAT programs. However, if your meal consists of at least 50% raw foods, in the form of, for example salads, then your body does not trigger the leukocytosis response.

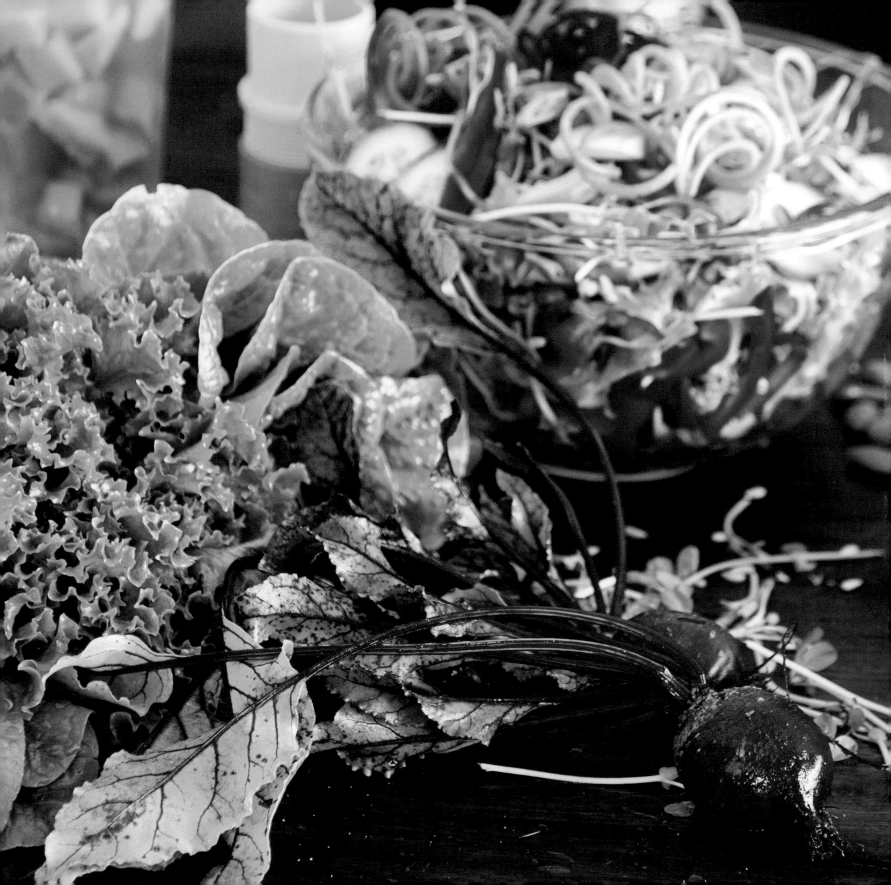

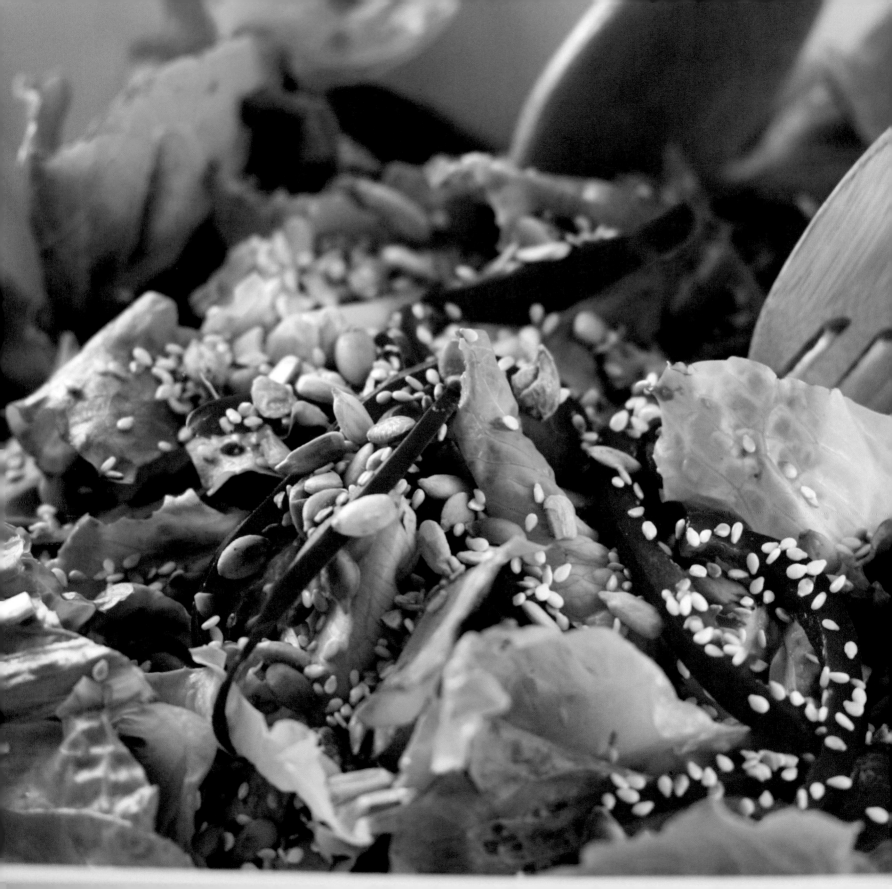

Crunchy Green Salad

Serves: 2
Preparation time: 15 minutes

Ingredients:
1 lettuce, washed and spun
½ cup grape tomatoes, sliced in half
1 small red capsicum (bell pepper), sliced thinly
1 avocado, peeled and cubed
1 Tbsp pepitas (pumpkin seeds)
1 Tbsp sunflower seeds
1 Tbsp sesame seeds
2 Tbsp flax seeds, ground

Method:
Place lettuce, tomatoes, capsicum and avocado in a medium sized salad bowl. Sprinkle with seeds and ground flax seeds. Serve with Gabriel Method Balsamic Salad Dressing (see page 200).

Greek Salad

Serves: 4
Preparation time: 10 minutes

Ingredients:
1 cucumber, sliced lengthways
2 roma tomatoes, sliced lengthways
1 small red onion, sliced lengthways
½ cup kalamata olives
125g feta cheese, cubed
¼ cup fresh basil leaves, shredded

Method:
1. Place all ingredients on a serving dish or in a salad bowl.
2. Serve with Gabriel Method Balsamic Dressing (see page 200).

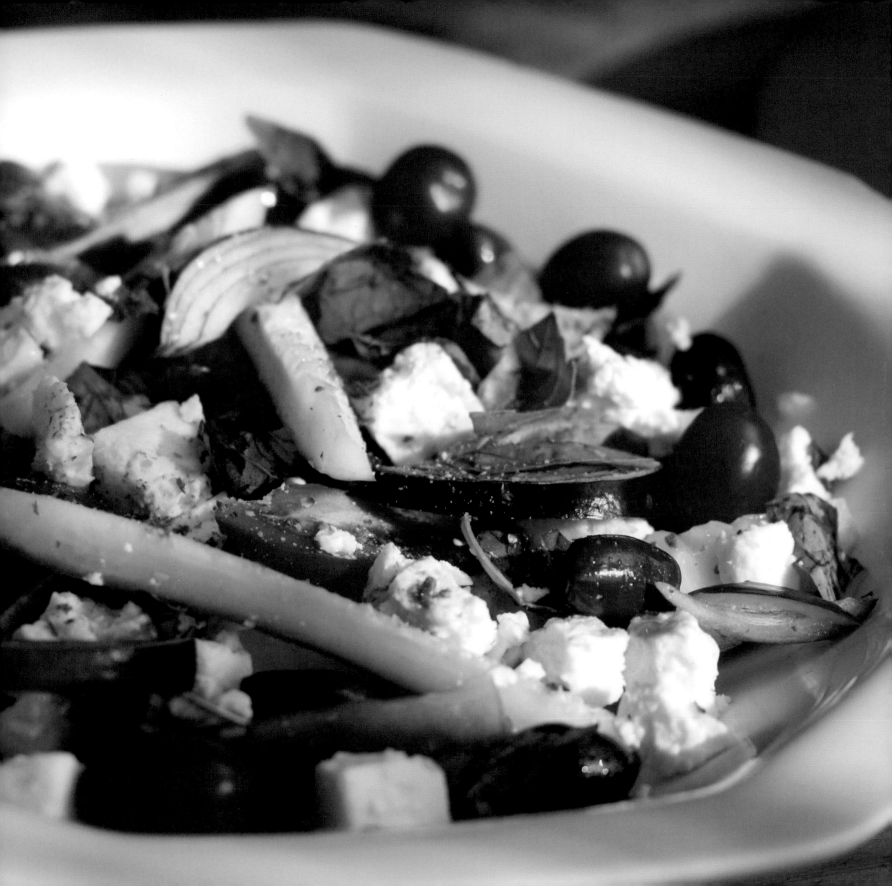

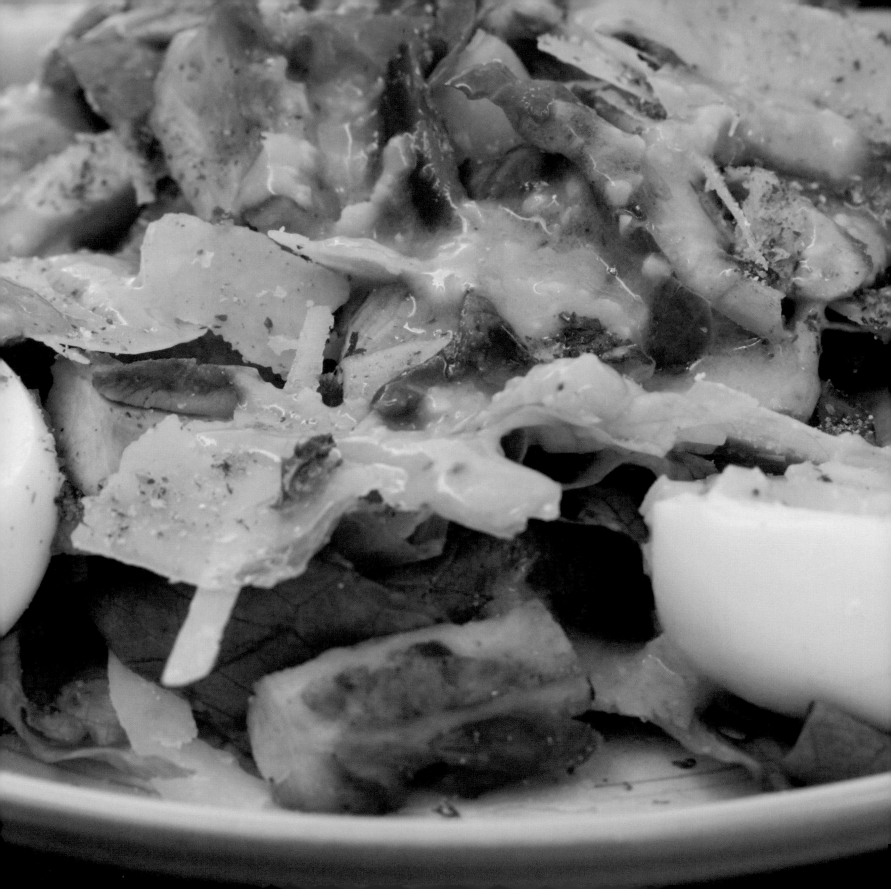

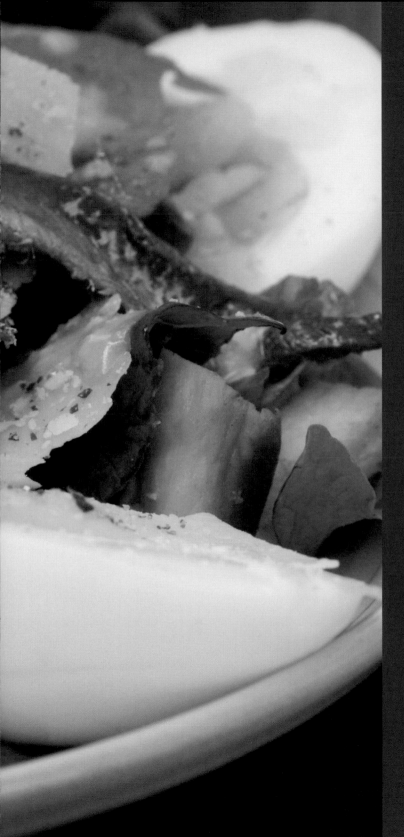

Chicken Caesar Salad

Serves: 2
Preparation time: 10 minutes
Cooking time: 10 minutes

Ingredients:
1 Tbsp Gabriel friendly cooking oil (see page 24)
400g chicken thigh fillets (organic, free range), cut into slices
10-20 cos lettuce (romaine) leaves, washed and dried
2 eggs (organic, free range), hard boiled, halved lengthways
½ cup Parmesan cheese, shaved
6 anchovies (optional)
2 Tbsp flax seeds, ground

Method:
1. Heat cooking oil in frying pan on medium heat. Cook chicken, stirring occasionally, until cooked through. Remove from pan with slotted spoon and set aside.
2. Place cos lettuce (romaine) leaves on serving plate(s). Top with cooked chicken, hard boiled eggs, shaved Parmesan and anchovies.
3. Serve with Caesar Dressing (see page 201).

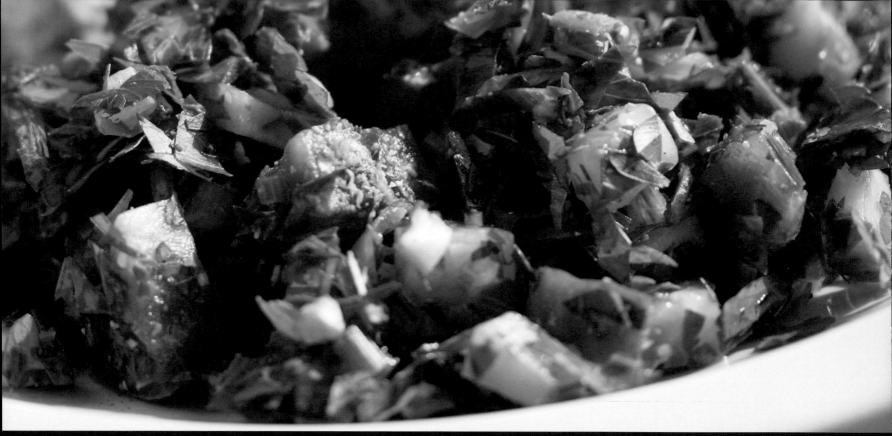

Tabouli

Serves: 4
Preparation time: 15 minutes

Ingredients:
3 roma tomatoes, cubed
3 spring onions (scallions), thinly sliced
1 Lebanese cucumber, cubed
4 cups parsley, coarsely chopped
⅔ cup mint, coarsely chopped
2 Tbsp flax seeds, ground

For the salad dressing:
80ml lemon juice
60ml olive oil
salt and pepper

Waldorf Salad

Serves: 6
Preparation time: 15 minutes

Ingredients:

3 apples, cubed
1 lemon, juiced
4 celery stalks, thinly sliced
1 avocado, cubed
1 cup walnuts, roughly chopped

2 Tbsp ground flax seeds
1 head of lettuce, washed, spun and cut.
⅓ cup Gabrielicious Mayonnaise (see page 202)
juice of half a lemon

Method:

1. Place apples and 2 Tbsp of lemon juice in a salad bowl. Toss to ensure apples are coated in juice. Add celery and walnuts. Add sliced lettuce leaves and avocado. Toss so that all ingredients are well combined.
2. Dress your salad with Gabriel Method Mayonnaise and remaining lemon juice.

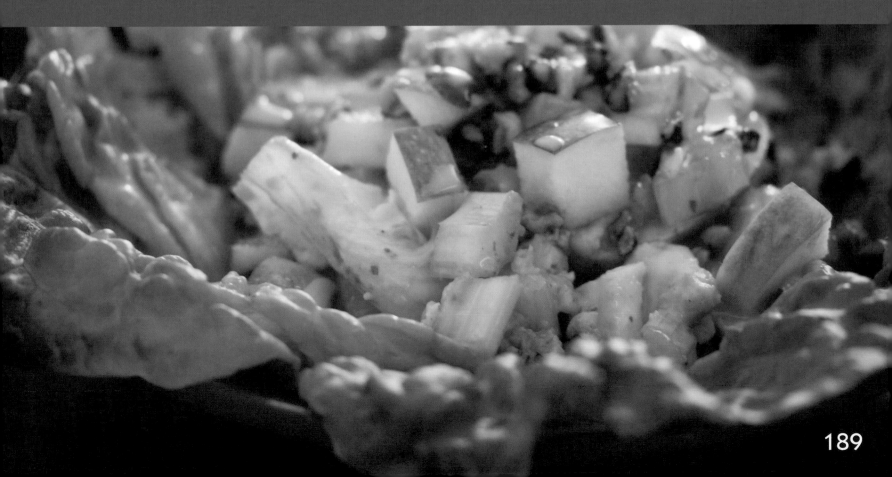

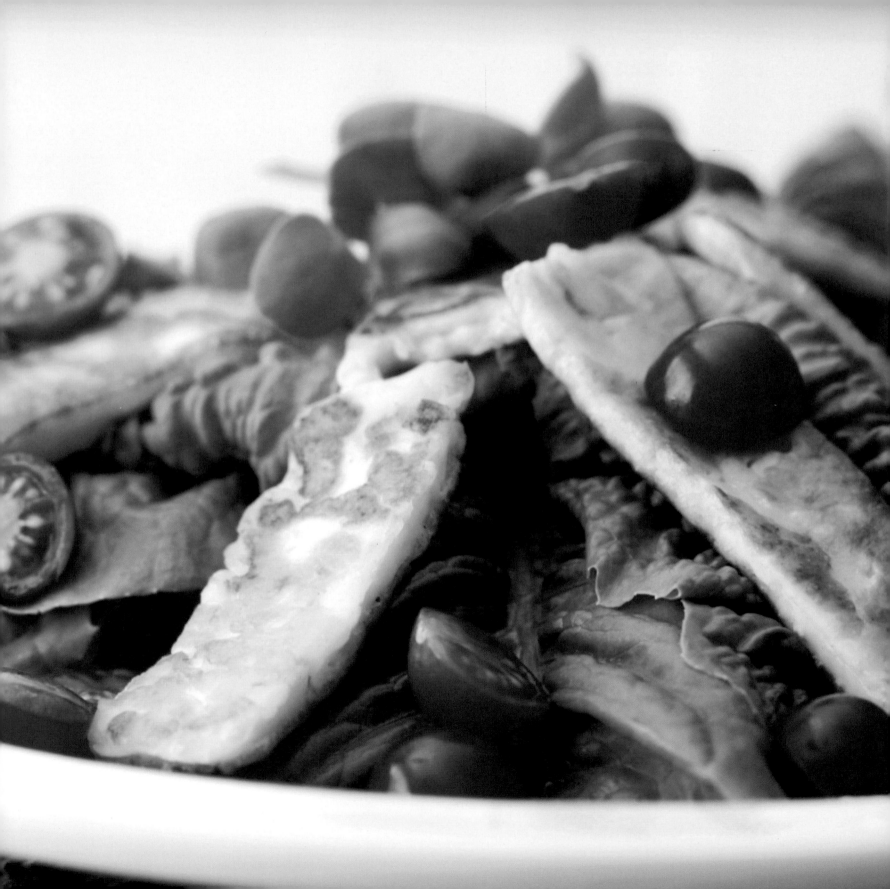

Simple Haloumi Salad

Serves: 2
Preparation time: 10 minutes
Cooking time: 5 minutes

Ingredients:
1 Tbsp Gabriel friendly cooking oil (see page 24)
180g haloumi cheese, sliced in 5mm strips
100g cherry tomatoes, halved
½ a cos lettuce (romaine), washed and spun
sunflower sprouts to serve

Method:
1. Heat cooking oil in a small frying pan on medium heat.
2. Place haloumi strips in hot pan. Cook on each side for 1-2 minutes or until the cheese is lightly browned.
3. Place washed cos leaves on a plate. Cover cos with haloumi strips, cherry tomatoes and sprouts.
4. Dress your salad with your home-made Gabriel Method Balsamic Dressing and sprinkle with flax seeds.
5. Dress your salad with home-made Gabrielicious Balsamic Dressing (see page 200).

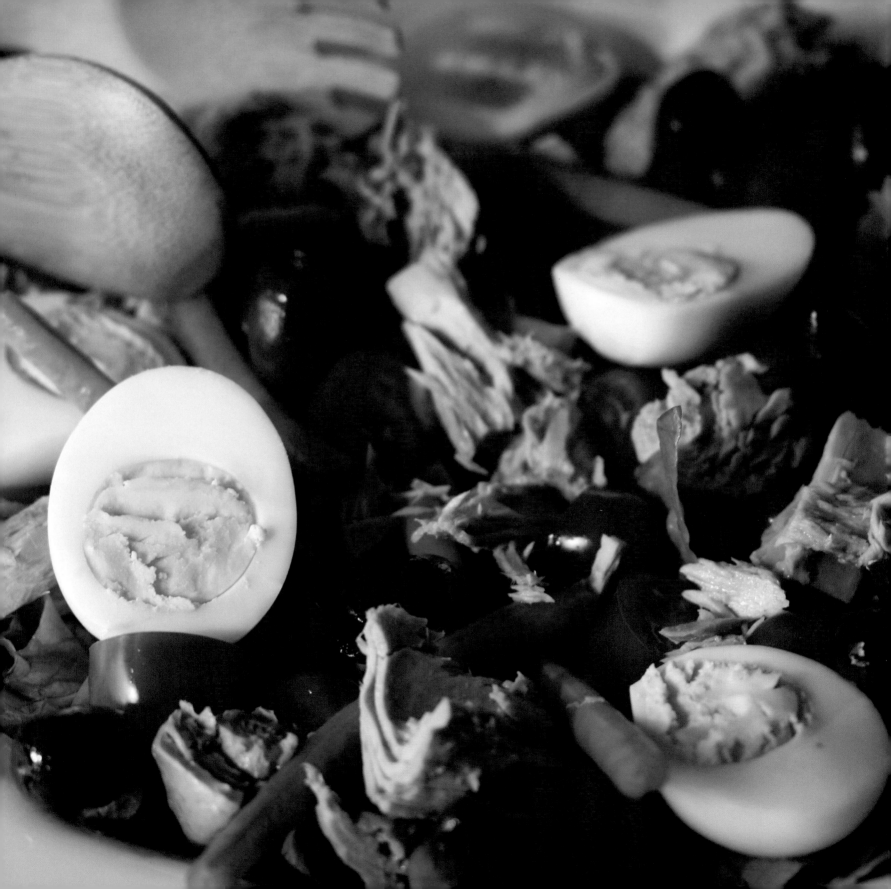

Salade Niçoise

Serves: 6
Preparation time: 20 minutes
Cooking time: 5 minutes

Ingredients:
450g green beans, lightly steamed
6 eggs (organic, free range), hard boiled, halved lengthways
250g cherry tomatoes, halved
1 cos lettuce (romaine), washed and spun
400g tuna
75g small black olives

Method:
1. On a large platter, place lettuce leaves. Arrange beans, tomatoes, eggs and tuna.

2. Drizzle with Salade Niçoise dressing (see page 205).

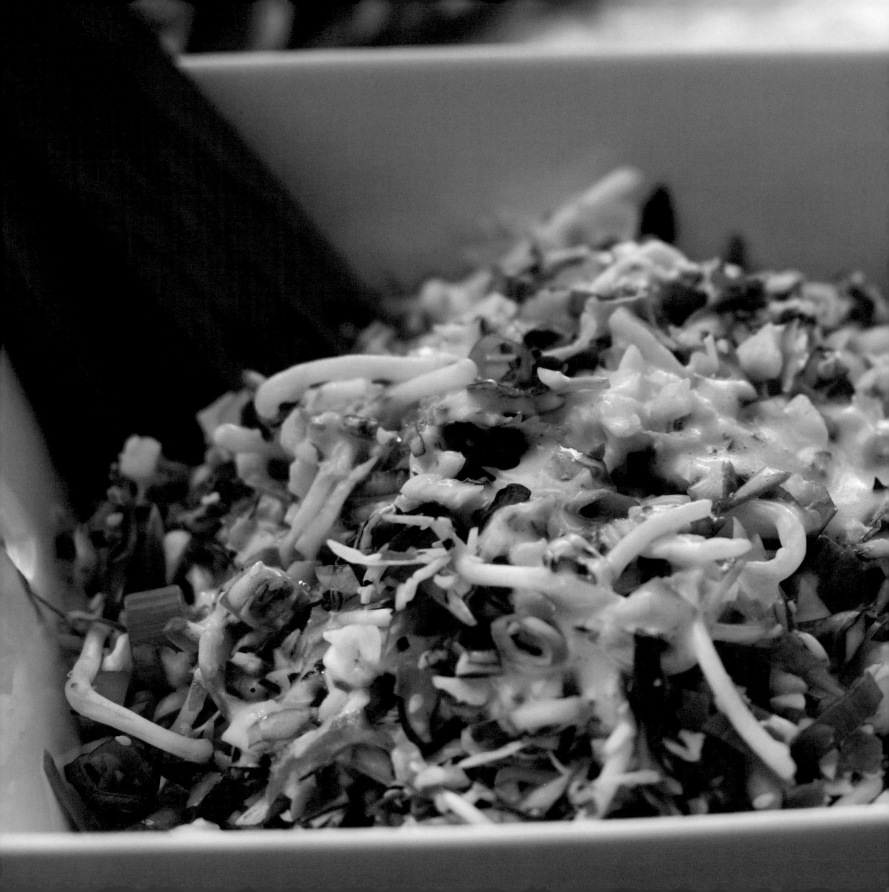

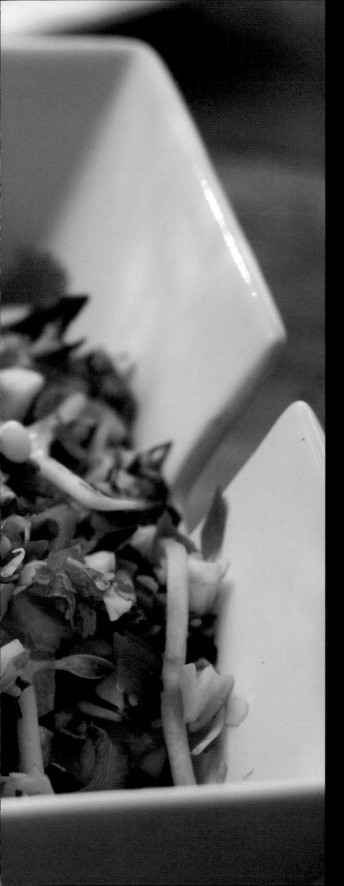

Sesame Coleslaw

Serves: 4
Preparation time: 20 minutes

Ingredients for the Salad:
¼ green cabbage, shredded
¼ red cabbage, shredded
1 carrot, grated
4 spring onions (scallions), thinly sliced
1 cup bean sprouts
1 Tbsp sesame seeds
⅓ cup fresh coriander, cut finely

Ingredients for the dressing:
¼ cup natural yoghurt
2 Tbsp Gabrielicious Mayonnaise (see page 202)
2 tsp paprika (or chilli powder)
¼ tsp xylitol
salt and pepper
1 tsp lime juice

Method:
1. In a medium sized bowl, place both types of cabbage, carrot, spring onions, bean sprouts, sesame seeds and coriander.
2. In a separate bowl place yoghurt, mayonnaise, paprika, xylitol and lime juice. Whisk until well combined. Add salt and pepper to taste.
3. Add dressing to coleslaw just prior to serving or alternatively, serve it on the side.

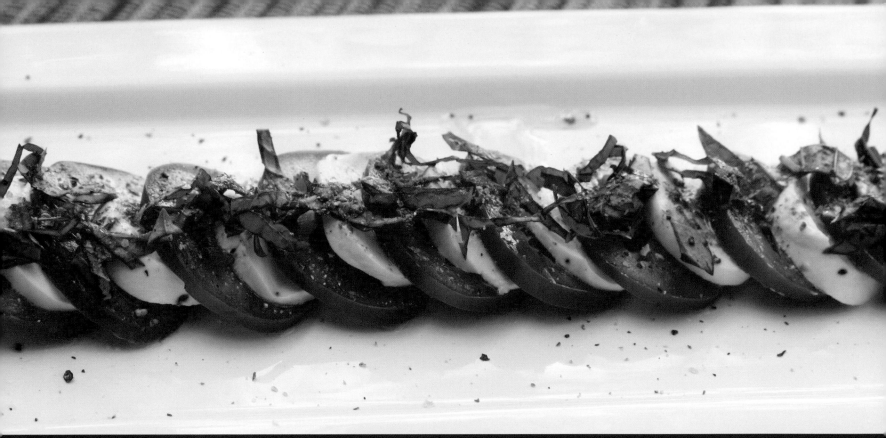

Tomato and Bocconcini

Serves: 4
Preparation time: 10 minutes

Ingredients:

4 roma tomatoes, sliced into rounds

150g bocconcini, sliced

¼ cup Gabrielicious cold oil (see page 23) or extra virgin cold pressed olive oil

2 tsp balsamic vinegar

¼ cup fresh basil leaves, shredded

1 Tbsp flax seeds, ground

Method:

1. Place the bocconcini and tomato slices on a serving platter, alternating tomato and bocconcini.
2. Drizzle the olive oil and balsamic vinegar over the top and scatter with the basil leaves.
3. Sprinkle with flax seeds prior to serving.

196

Baby Spinach and Goat's Cheese Salad

Serves: 4
Preparation time: 10 minutes

Ingredients:
4 handfuls baby spinach leaves
2 Tbsp pine nuts, lightly toasted in frying pan, no oil required
1 avocado, sliced thinly
80g goat's cheese, chopped into small pieces
2 Tbsp ground flax seeds

Method:
1. Place all ingredients in salad bowl.
2. Dress with Gabriel Method Balsamic Dressing (see page 200) and sprinkle with flax seeds.

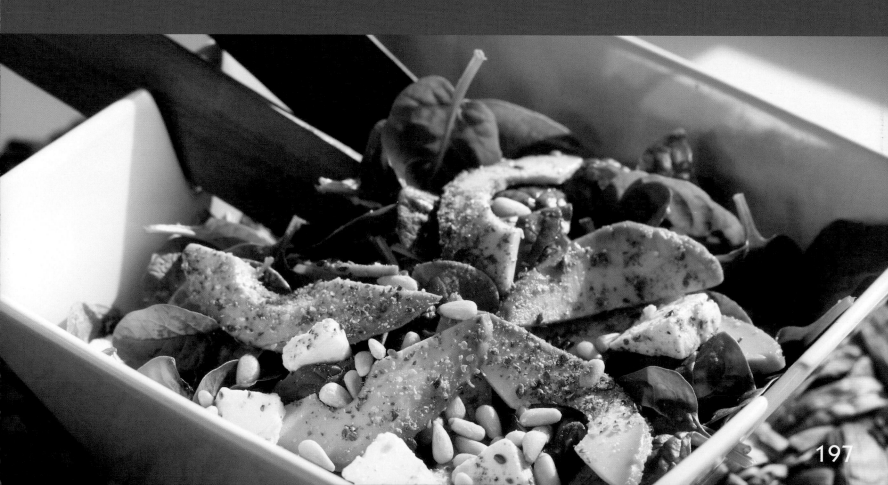

Healthy dressings are some of the easiest ways that you can get those essential Omega-3s.

Cold-pressed flaxseed, chia seed and walnut oil are all rich in Omega-3s. If you find that you don't like the flavour of these oils – and admittedly some take a little getting used to – then use olive oil and try blending it with the Omega-3 rich oils until you find the right proportion that works for you.

Try incorporating apple cider vinegar into your salad dressings for the added flavour and health properties it has to offer.

Experiment, knowing that your taste may eventually change and you'll actually start to crave more and more of these marvelous oils.

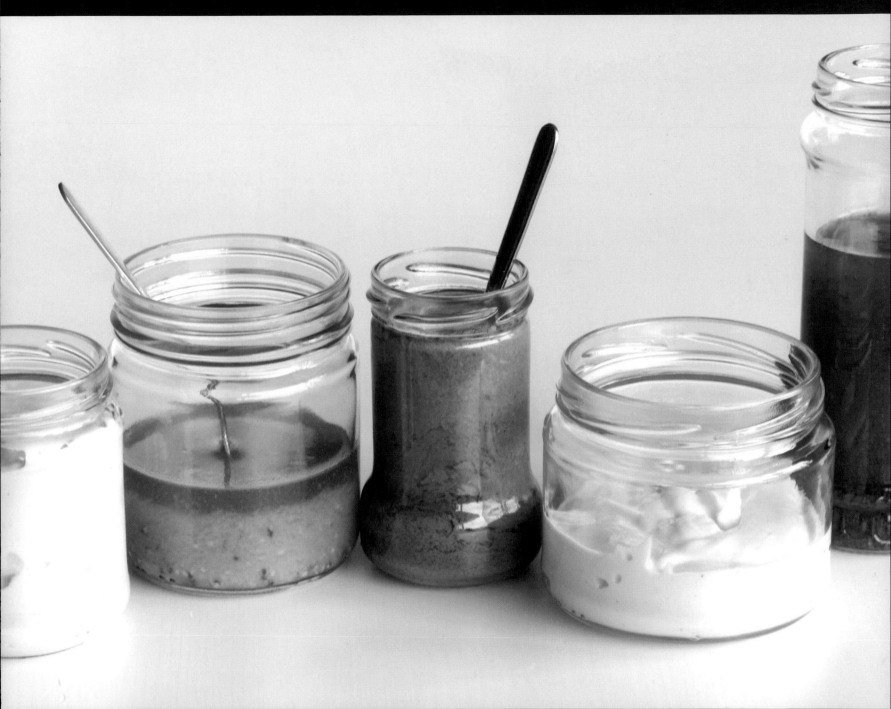

Balsamic Salad Dressing

Makes: 250 mls
Preparation time: 5 minutes

Ingredients:
¼ cup balsamic vinegar
¾ cup Gabrielicious cold oil (see page 23) or
extra virgin cold pressed olive oil
1½ tsp Dijon mustard
1 Tbsp lemon juice
1 garlic clove, peeled, crushed
salt and pepper

Method:
1. Place all ingredients into a jar. Tighten jar lid and shake thoroughly until well combined.
2. Add to your salad just prior to serving or simply place dressing jar on the table for people to dress their own salad.
3. Store in the refridgerator, take out 10 minutes prior to serving and shake well.

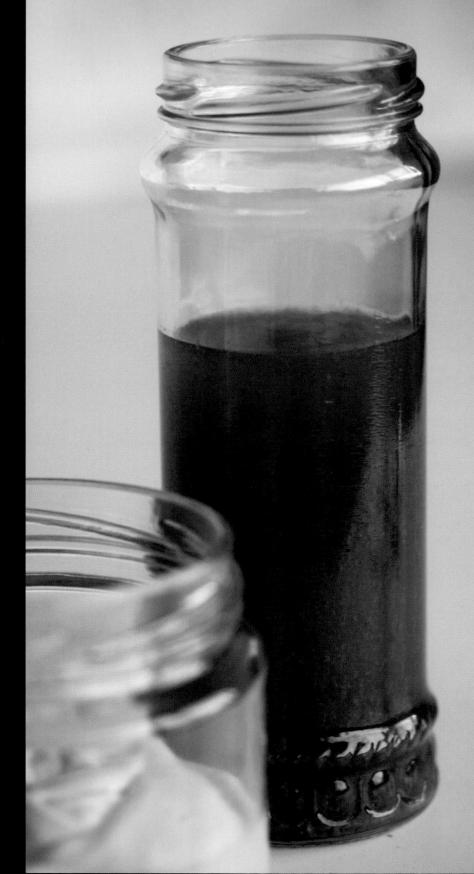

Caesar Dressing

Makes: 150ml
Preparation time: 10 minutes

Ingredients:
1 egg yolk
2 tsp Dijon mustard
1 garlic clove
2 Tbsp lemon juice
3 anchovies
¼ cup Parmesan cheese
½ cup Gabrielicious cold oil
(see page 23) or extra virgin
cold pressed olive oil

Method:
1. Combine all ingredients, except oil, using a food processor or stick blender. Add oil gradually, a little at a time, until you achieve a smooth and creamy consistency.
2. Drizzle over your salad prior to serving, sprinkle with flax seeds and enjoy!

201

Gabrielicious Mayonnaise

Makes: 175mls
Preparation time: 10 minutes

Ingredients:
2 egg yolks
1 tsp Dijon mustard
1 Tbsp white wine vinegar
1 Tbsp lemon juice
1 Tbsp of lemon juice
½ cup Gabrielicious cold oil
(see page 23) or extra virgin cold
pressed olive oil
healthy salt (see page 17)
pepper to taste

Method:
1. Combine egg yolks, mustard and vinegar.
2. Gradually add oil, a small amount at a time. Whisk until well combined before adding more oil. Once all oil has been added, mix for a few seconds with a stick blender to achieve a thick and creamy conistency.
3. Add salt and pepper to taste.
4. Can be refrigerated for up to 2 days.

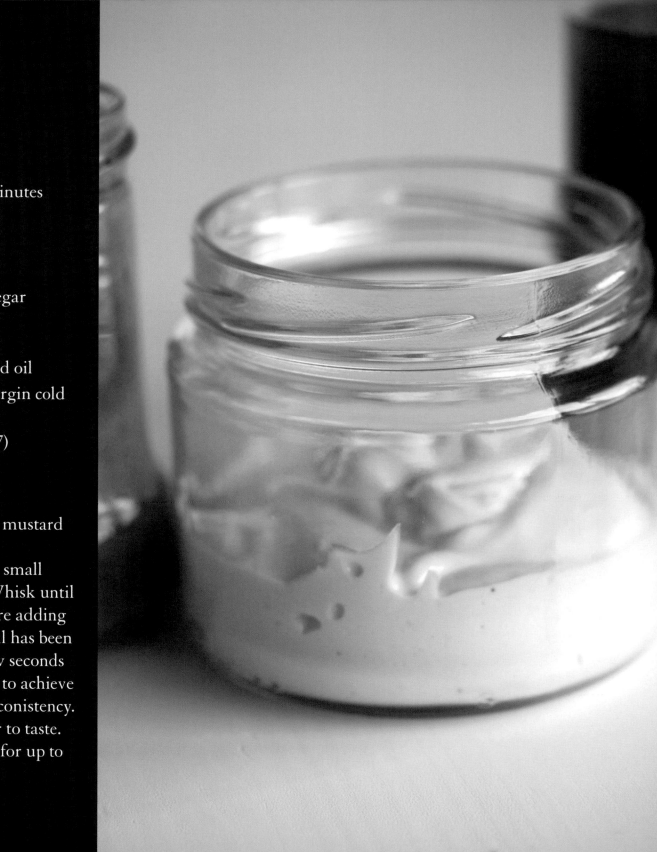

Honey Mustard Dressing

Makes: 175 mls
Preparation time: 10 minutes

Ingredients:

1 tsp grain mustard

1 tsp raw unprocessed honey

2 Tbsp white wine vinegar

125ml Gabrielicious cold oil (see page 23) or extra virgin cold pressed olive oil

salt and pepper

1 Tbsp parsley (optional)

Method:

1. Place mustard, honey, vinegar, olive oil, salt and pepper in a jar. Tighten jar lid and shake thoroughly until well combined.
2. Add parsley prior to serving.
3. Add to your salad just prior to serving or place dressing jar on the table for people to dress their own salad!

Chilli Tahini Sauce

Makes: 150ml
Preparation time: 5 minutes

Ingredients:
¼ cup Balsamic vinegar
2 Tbsp tahini
70ml Gabrielicious cold oil
(see page 23) or extra virgin cold
pressed olive oil
1 Tbsp lemon juice
¼ tsp chilli powder, vary
according to taste

Method:
Place all ingredients in a glass
jar. Put lid on tight and shake
until well combined.

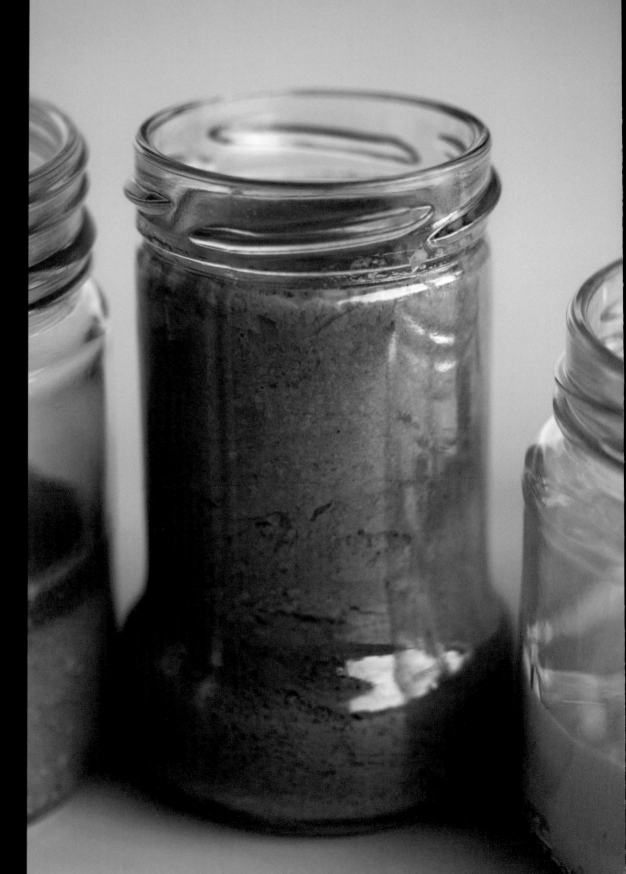

Niçoise Dressing

Makes: 200 mls
Preparation time: 10 minutes

Ingredients:
1 Tbsp flax seeds, ground
1 spring onion, finely chopped
1 clove garlic, crushed
1 tsp Dijon mustard
1 Tbsp white wine vinegar
1 Tbsp lemon juice
⅔ cup Gabrielicious cold oil (see page 23) or
extra virgin cold pressed olive oil
¼ cup basil leaves
salt & pepper to season

Method:
1. Process all ingredients in a food processor until the mixture is well combined.
2. Season to taste with salt, pepper and xylitol.

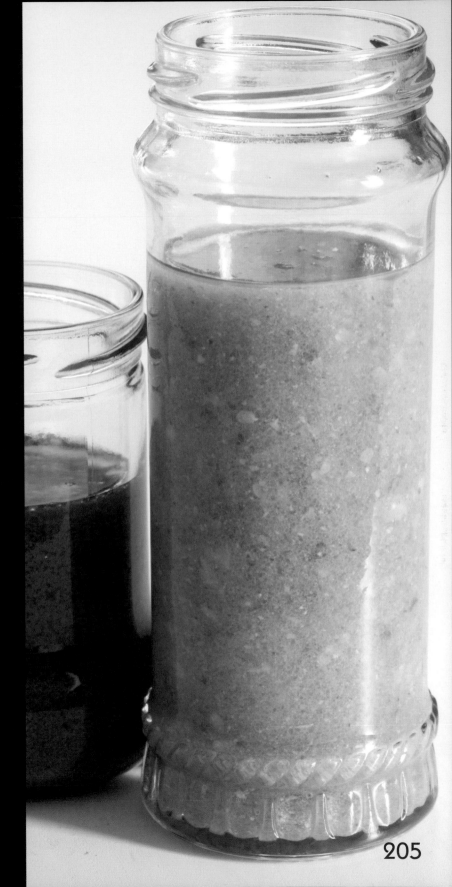

205

Makes: 120 mls
Preparation time: 10 minutes

Ingredients:

½ cup tomato paste

2½ tsp xylitol

2 tsp salt

2 tsp white wine vinegar

Method:

1. Place all ingredients together in bowl. Mix well to combine.
2. Either place in small bowl with teaspoon to serve or pour into recycled squeeze bottle.

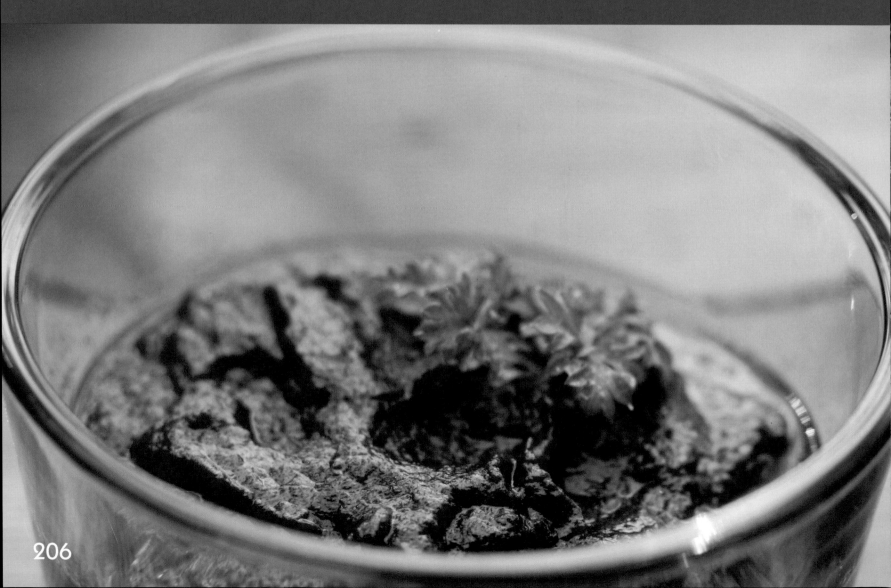

Chilli Tomato Sauce

Follow the Gabriel Method Tomato Sauce recipe adding two teaspoons of chilli powder for a mild sauce, or more if you like it hot. Stir and enjoy!

Fresh, Live Juices

Vegetable juices are a great way of getting a quick dose of vitality. Juicing breaks down the cellular walls of the vegetables, allowing the full complement of nutrition to become instantly available to your digestive system. This convenience can come at a cost because the concentration of nutrition is a little like having too much of a good thing too fast. Pure carrot juice, beet root and most fruit juices, elevate your blood sugar way too quickly. Celery and Swiss chard (silverbeet) stabilise blood sugar. So a mixture of 60% celery and or Swiss chard with fruits and other vegetables provides the right balance. Having your juice with a Gabriel Method meal will not only ease your appetite and maintain blood sugar levels, it will provide additional nutrition and enzymes for digestion.

Slow-pressing, masticating juice extractors are best. High-speed extractors tend to heat the juice, partially cooking it and also aerating it, helping to speed up oxidisation thus turning juices brown and unpalatable while also compromising their nutritional value.

Slow pressing, masticating juicers are more expensive, but they're well worth the investment. They're incredibly versatile in that they can extract wheatgrass juice, make fruit sorbets as well as nut milks and butters.

Nevertheless, high speed juicers can be used as long as the juice is consumed immediately so that the nutritional loss is minimal.

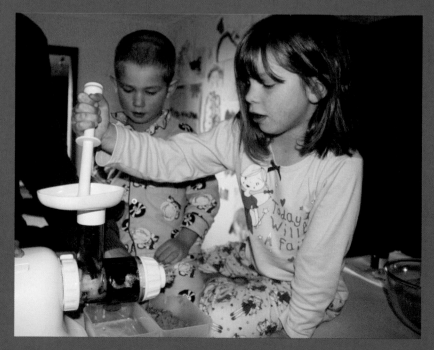

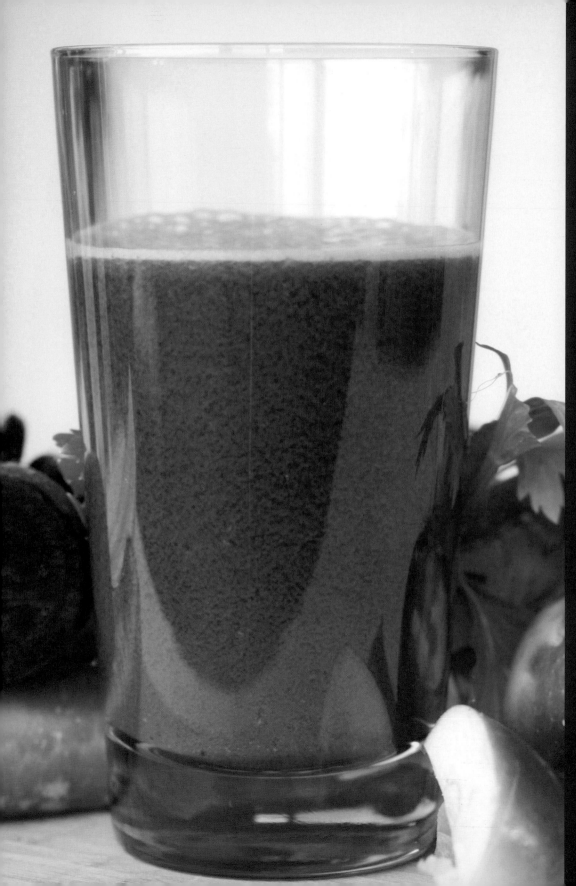

Sample Super Vitality Blood Cleansing Juice

Ingredients:
2-3 celery stalks
1 large silverbeet (Swiss chard) leaf
1 carrot
1 apple
1 clove garlic
1 thin slice of ginger

Method:
Run all ingredients through a slow-pressing, masticating juice extractor. Serve immediately.

Grow Your Own

Get the Family Involved

Losing weight the Gabriel Method way is much easier if you can get the family involved. Children especially like the idea of gardening and growing their own food. So, if you have the space for it, growing your own food can be one of the most satisfying and fun contributions you can make to your weightloss efforts. Growing the food as a family is also a lot of fun. Even young children can help water plants and pick your happily grown produce.

Growing Your Own

There are so many reasons to grow your own: you know exactly where your food has come from, you have access to the freshest produce you could possibly have, it tastes amazing and it's what your body craves on a nutritional level. By loving and nourishing your plants, you are loving and nourishing yourself. You and your family get to witness the wonders of real foods coming to life and all the colours and forms they take along the way. But most of all, there is nothing more satisfying than going out to your garden to pick your own grown produce to prepare your meal with!

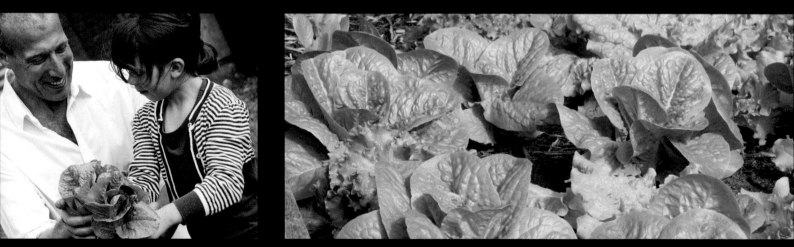

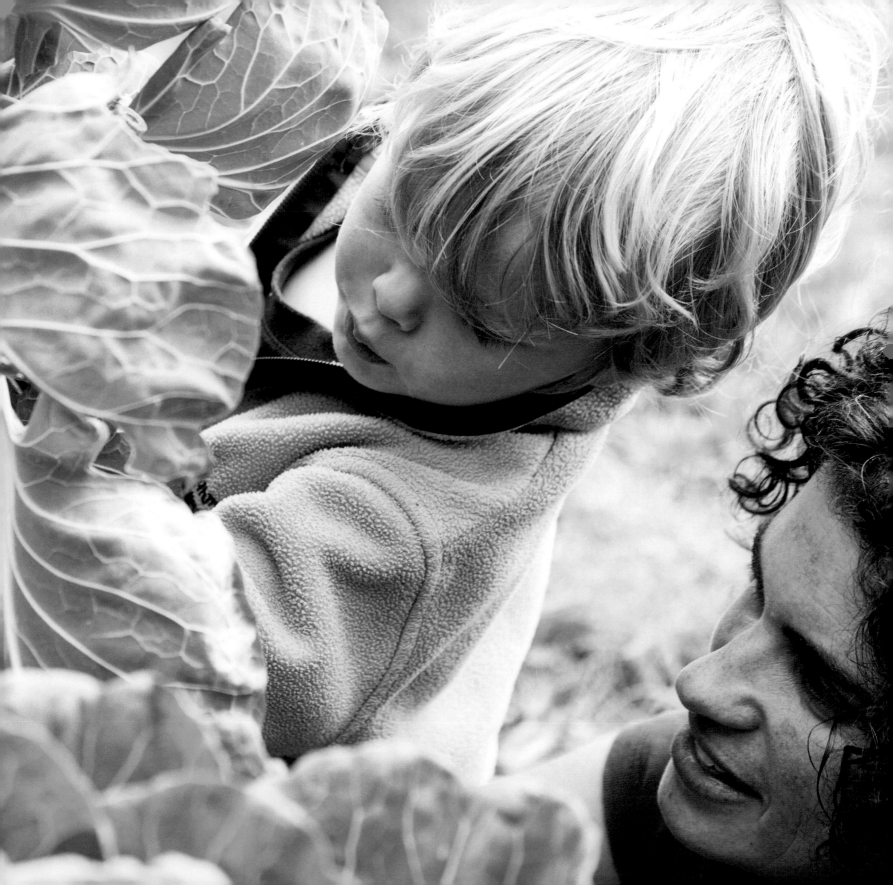

Sprouting

Growing Sprouts

If you have a sprouter, it's best to follow the manufacturer's instructions. If not, you can achieve the same results with a glass jar and clean tea towel or cheese cloth.

You can buy seeds online or purchase organic seed mixes from your favourite health food shop. Either way, make sure your seeds are organic. Experiment with different nuts and seeds to find which ones you like best.

Basic sprouting instructions:

1. Rinse your seeds in a sieve and pick out any that are off-colour, broken or mouldy.
2. Fill ⅓ of a jar with seeds and top up with water. Tie the tea towel to the top of the jar using an elastic band or string. Allow to soak for 4-12 hours, depending on which seeds or nuts you are sprouting. As a general rule, small, softer seeds need less soaking time, say 4 hours, whereas larger, harder nuts may need up to 12 hours. Rinse the seeds and change the water every few hours while they are soaking.
3. Drain your seeds of water. Rinse them and turn the jar upside down while propped at an angle for drainage. Keep out of direct sunlight and in an area that is relatively stable in temperature.
4. Rinse at least once a day until you eat them. They are generally considered ready when the root has grown to the approximate length of the sprouted seed. Store in fridge, rinsing every day or two. The sooner you eat your sprouts the better, though they can keep up to a week in the fridge with regular rinsing.

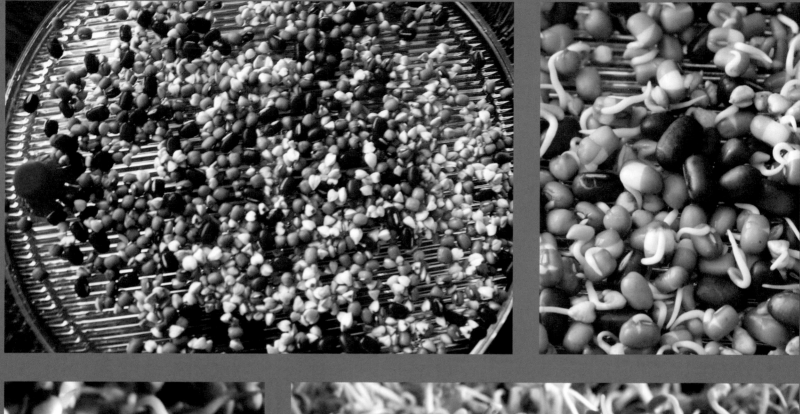

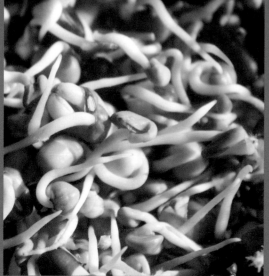

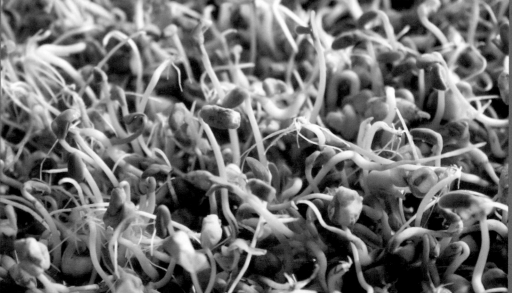

Wheatgrass

Wheatgrass juice is the most powerful all-round superfood that you can get. Highly nutritious and life-force dense, it's also a powerful cleanser and detoxifier. If you have little bit of space and time, you can grow your own. It's easy and tremendously satisfying.

Alternatively do a little research, starting with your health food shop, to see if someone local is growing it by the tray. You can then contract with them to grow several trays of wheatgrass for you every week. Cut the grass as you need it and extract your own juice. This is what I do when I don't have the time to grow my own.

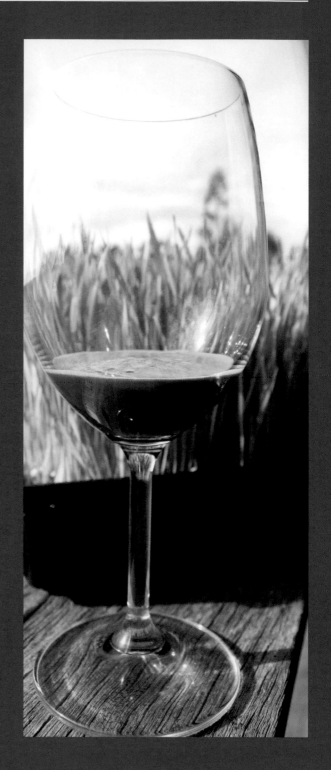

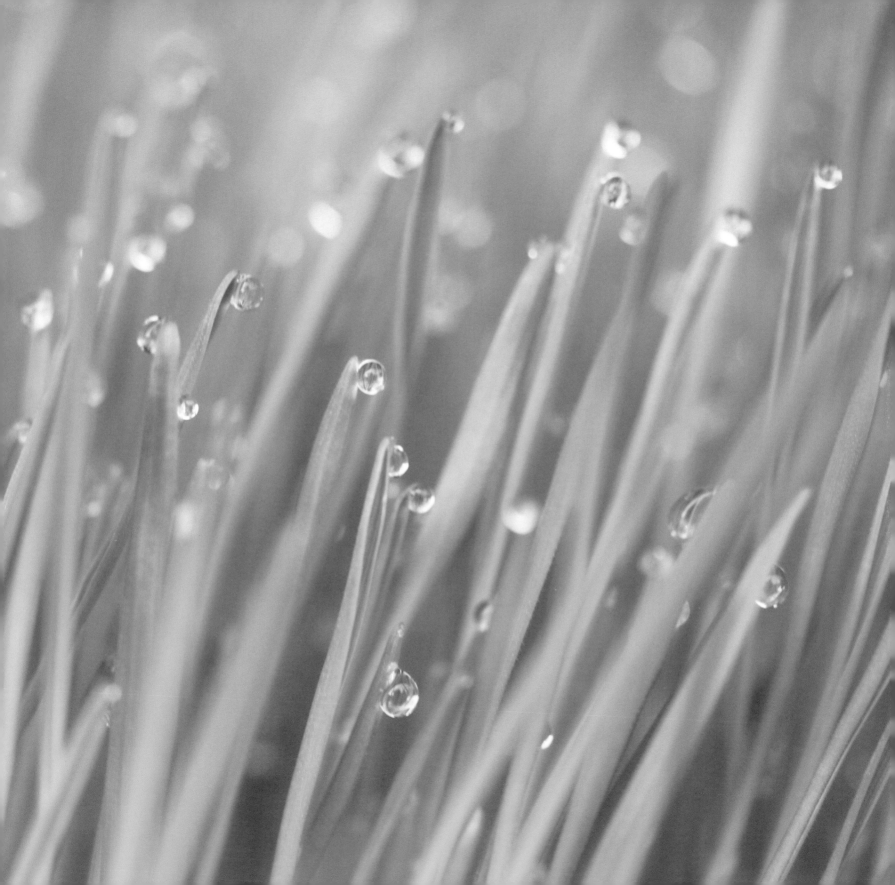

Growing Wheatgrass

Things you will need:
- organic wheat grains
- soaking container e.g. baking dish
- wheatgrass growing tray: approximately 20cm width, 30cm length, 5cm depth with drainage holes at base
- unbleached butchers paper
- organic potting mix or soil
- unbleached cloth

Easy steps to growing your own Wheatgrass:
1. Place your organic wheat seeds into a baking dish, or similar, and cover with water. Soak seeds overnight.
2. Wash and rinse grain until the water runs clear. Dampen the soil with a spray bottle.
3. Prepare your growing tray by placing unbleached butchers paper at the base. This will prevent soil loss. Fill your tray approximately ¾ full with organic potting mix or soil.
4. Spread your sprouted wheat seeds over the top, try to cover all the soil with seeds while avoiding having the seeds overlap each other.
5. Water your seeds thoroughly and cover with unbleached cloth. Leave in a dark place for 2-3 days.
6. Uncover your seeds and place in a light area sheltered from wind and rain, birds and rodents. Water daily until wheatgrass is mature and ready to juice.
7. The best way to juice your wheatgrass is with a slow turning wheatgrass juicer or hand juicer. Cut your wheatgrass with scissors and feed it through your juicer. One serve of wheatgrass is approximately 30ml.

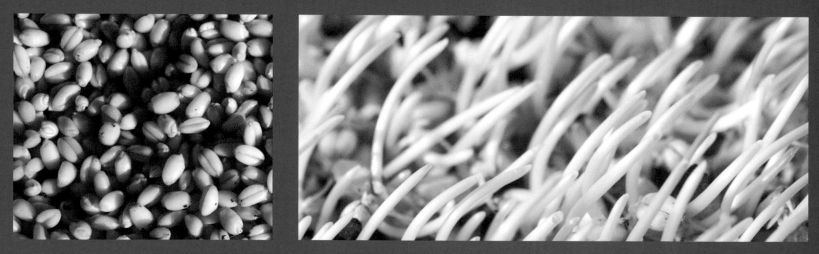

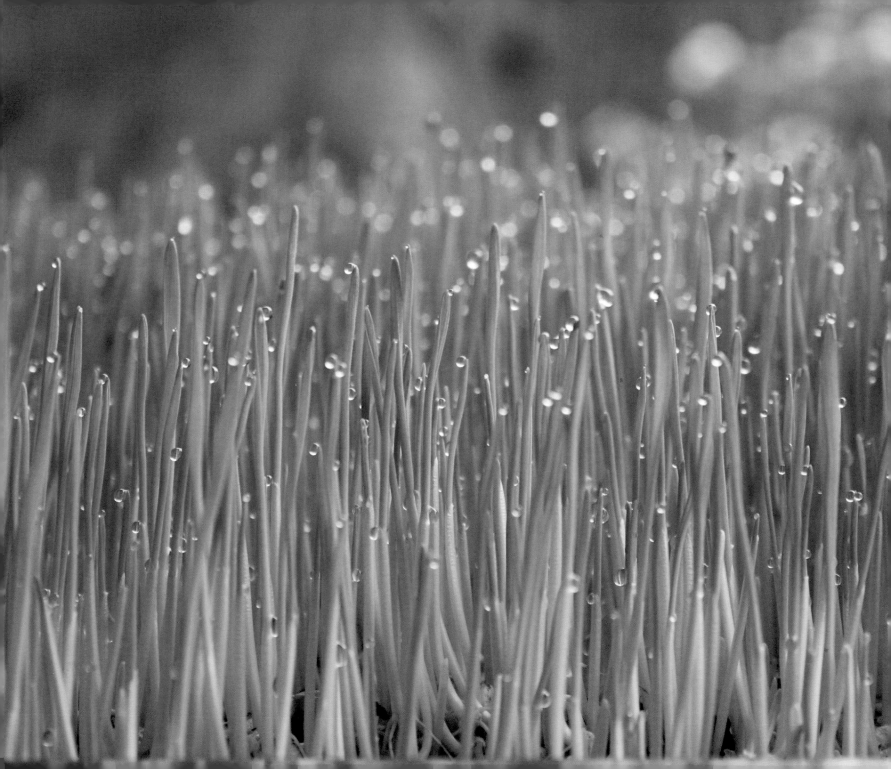

Drinks and Desserts

When it comes to weightloss, it's not about calories in and calories out. It's all about the hormonal response that your body has to the foods that you put into it.

The dessert recipes that we've included here might surprise you. Some of them sound fattening and some of them certainly look fattening.

Instead, our recipes are nutritionally dense and more importantly, the ingredients that we use and the combinations and proportions that they are in will mean that your body's hormonal response to them will result in blood sugar stabilisation that will, in turn, help turn off the FAT programs.

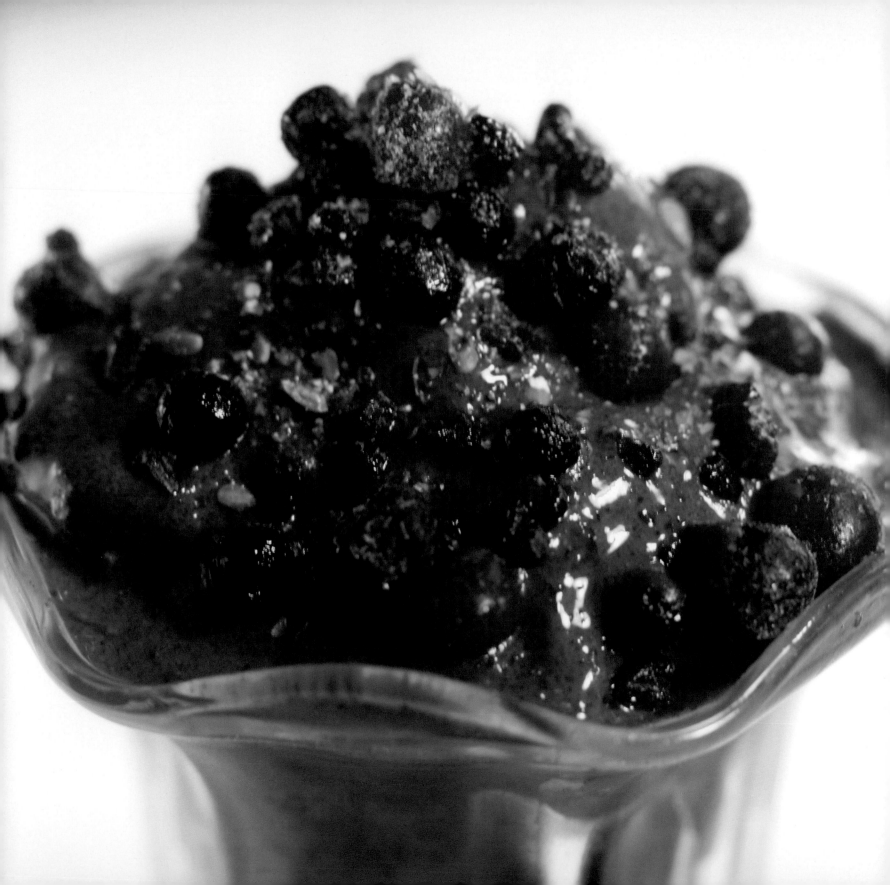

Drinks and Desserts

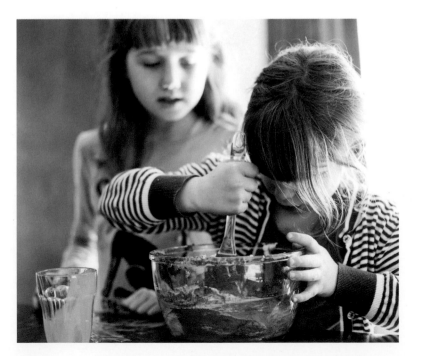

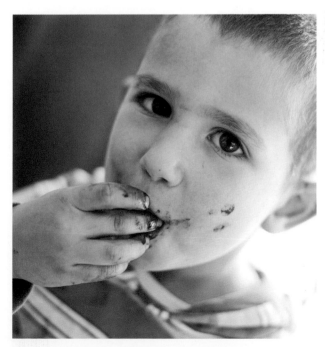

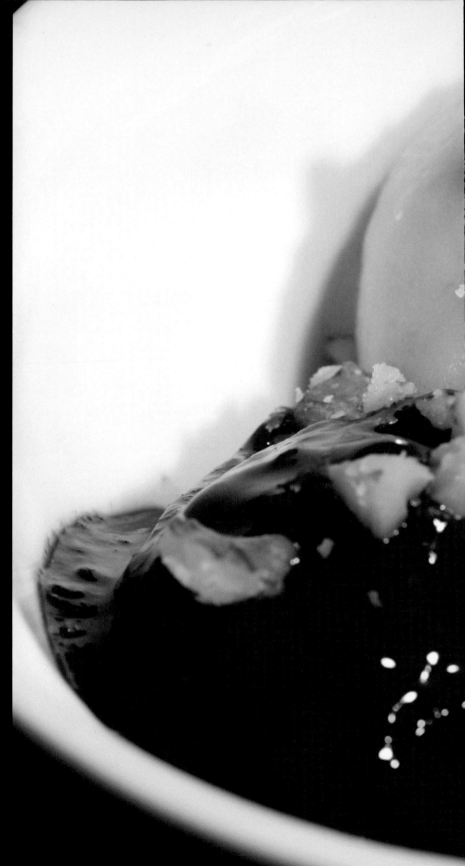

"On the following pages you will find healthy delicious alternatives to ice cream made from fruit, yoghurt and healthy sweeteners. Fast, easy, healthy, tasty.... what more can we say? And the kids love it! Gabriel Method at its finest.

If you have a macerating juicer these sorbets couldn't be easier to make. We recommend investing in one – it's worth it. But, if you add frozen bananas to the mix and use a stick blender the result is and just as good."

100% Fruit Ice Cream

Serves: 2
Preparation time: 5 minutes

Ingredients:
2 cups of your choice of frozen fruit
Some of our favourites include: mango, blueberry, strawberry, passionfruit and banana.

Method:
Set your juicer up so the ice cream nozzle is on. Feed the frozen fruit through, into the juicer pushing it through with the plunger until all has gone through. Distribute ice cream into 2 bowls and serve (sprinkled with flax seeds for extra goodness).

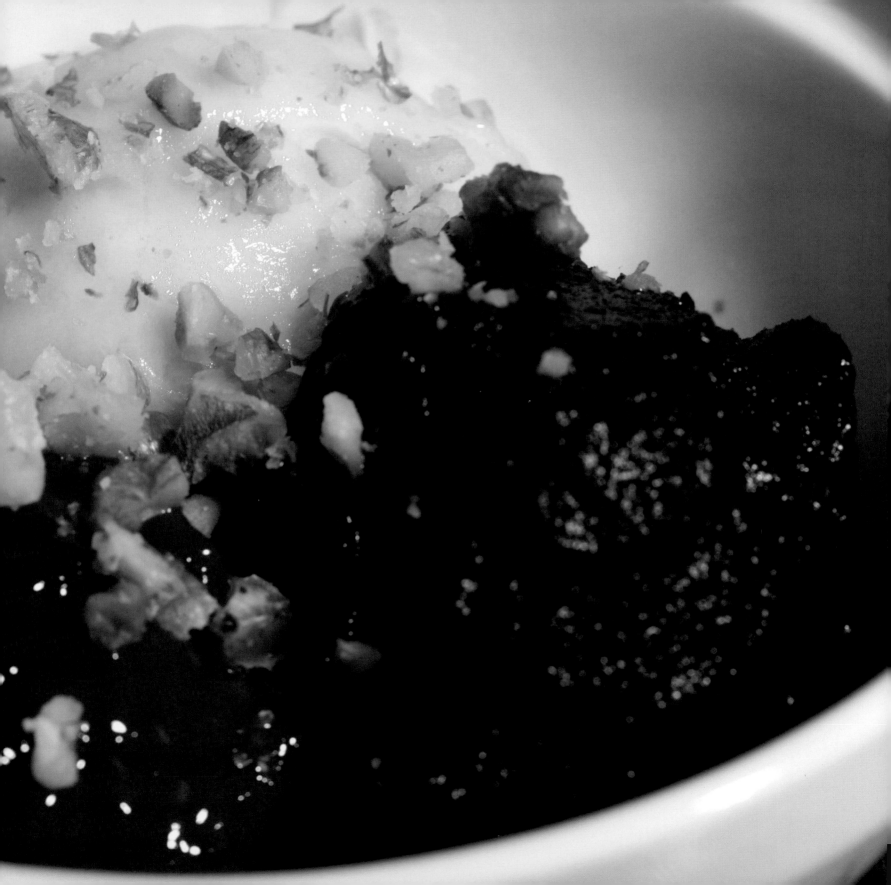

Fruity Flax Pops

Serves: 4 icypoles
Preparation time: 5 minutes
Setting time: 3 hours, minimum

Variations:
Strawberry Flax Pop:
1 cup yoghurt
8 strawberries, halved
1 Tbsp flax seeds, ground
1 Tbsp protein powder
a pinch of stevia

Kiwi Pop:
1 kiwi fruit
1 Tbsp flax seeds, ground

Passionfruit Flax Pop:
1 cup yoghurt
8 Tbsp passionfruit pulp (1-2 passionfruits)
1 Tbsp flax seeds, ground
1 Tbsp protein powder
a pinch of stevia

Pineapple Pop:
400g pineapple, chopped into pieces
1 Tbsp flax seeds, ground

Method:
1. Place ingredients of your chosen flavour in a mixing jug. Blend together with stick blender.
2. Pour mixture into icy pole (popsicle) moulds and freeze for 3 hours or until set.

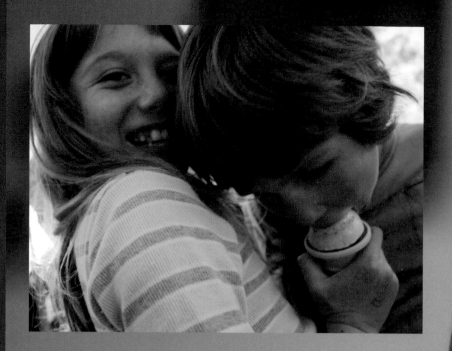

"These are fun, colourful snacks that kids will love as an after school treat or when in need of an energy boost."

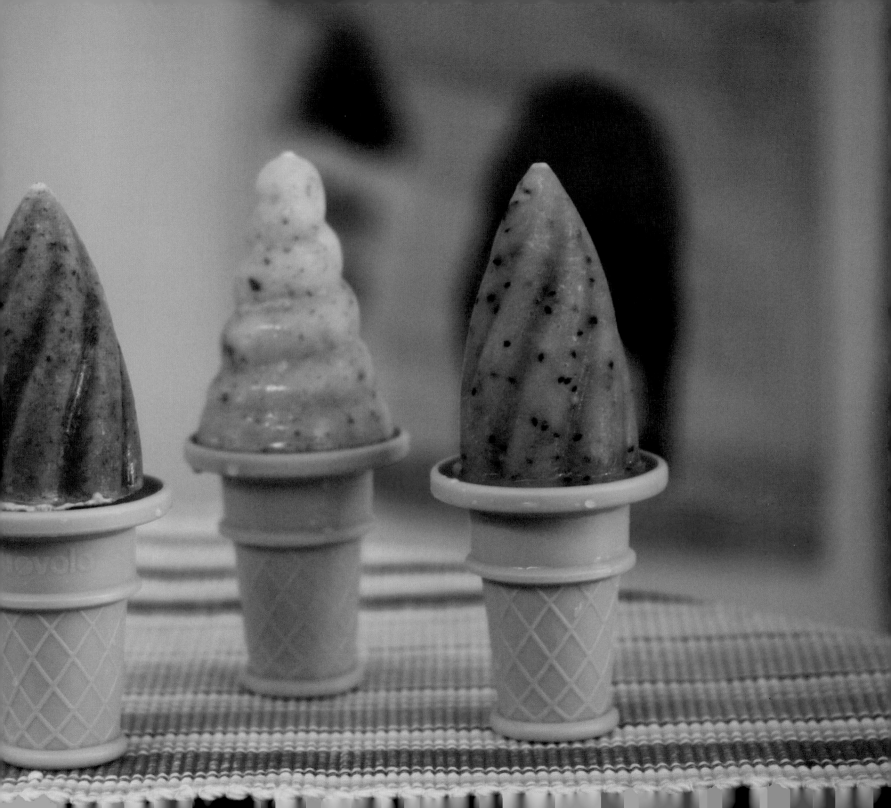

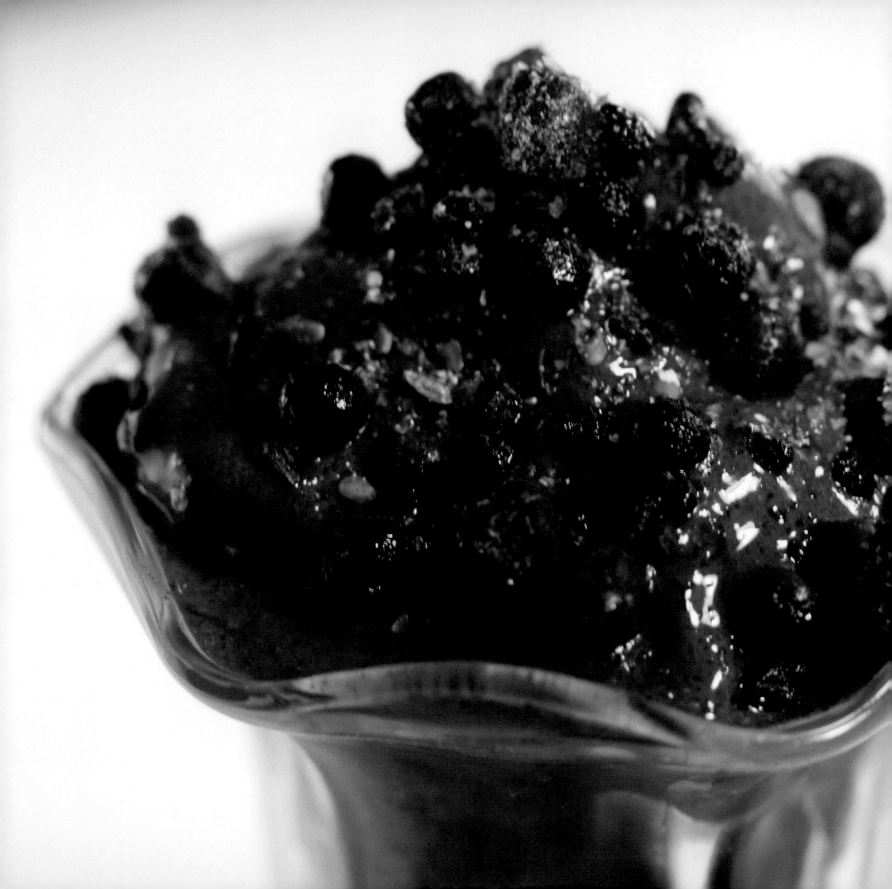

Easy Fruit Ice Cream

Serves: 4 kiddy size
Preparation time: 5 minutes

Ingredients:
⅔ cup plain yoghurt
¾ cup of your chosen frozen fruit
1 Tbsp flax seeds, ground
a pinch of stevia (recommended for raspberries or mixed berries, other fruits are naturally sweet enough)
contents of 1 probiotic and 1 digestive enzyme capsule (optional)

Optional flavours:
mango
blueberry
strawberry
passionfruit

Method:
1. Place yoghurt and 1 cup of your choice of frozen fruit into a blending jug. If the fruit is very hard, allow it to soften for a few minutes. Fruit should be in small pieces rather than a frozen block.
2. Mix together using a stick blender. Distribute among 4 bowls, sprinkle with flax seeds and serve.

Freezing Your Fruit
- Always peel bananas before freezing. Make sure that they are very ripe prior to freezing, otherwise that bitter unripe banana taste will dominate in your creations. Place in airtight freezer container.
- For mangoes, cut lengthways on either side of seed. Scoop fruit out of skin using a dessert spoon. Place in airtight freezer container.
- For passionfruit pulp, freeze into an ice cube tray to avoid creating one large block.

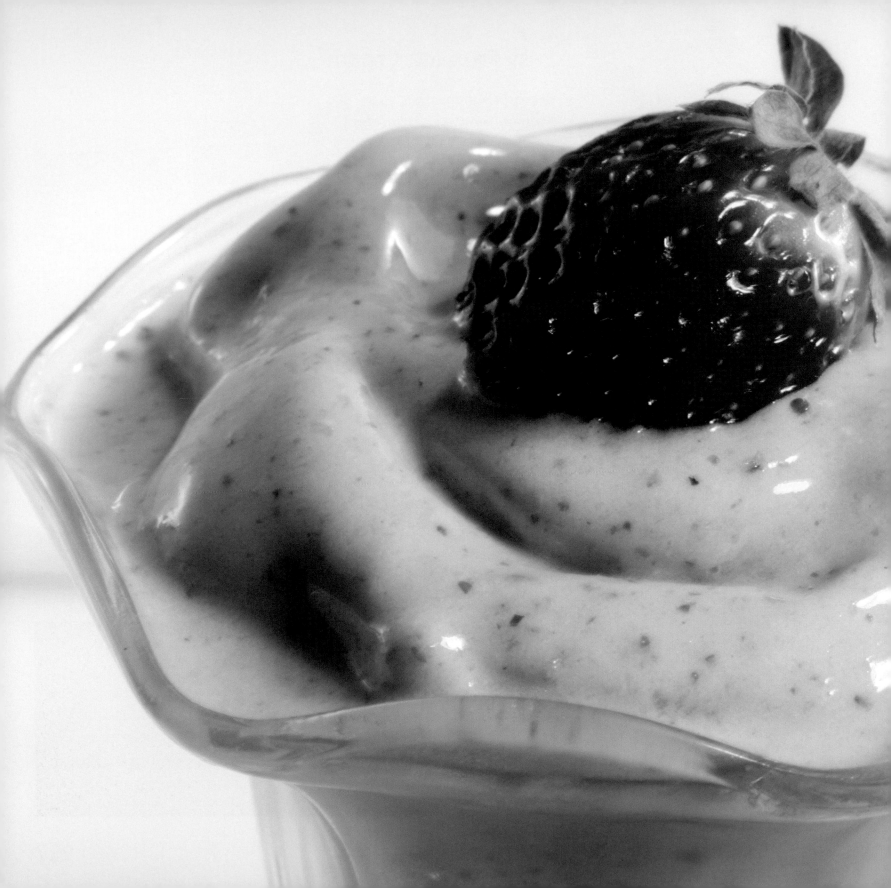

Easy Vanilla Ice Cream

Serves: 2 kiddy serves
Preparation time: 5 minutes

Ingredients:
2 bananas, frozen, chopped
¼ cup milk, preferably Gabriel Method Nut Milk
(see page 256)
1 tsp vanilla essence
1 Tbsp flax seeds, ground
2 tsp protein powder
contents of 1 probiotic and 1 digestive enzyme capsule
(optional)

Method:
Place all ingredients in mixing jug. Blend together with
stick blender, ensuring all banana pieces are thoroughly
mixed through. Serve immediately.

Easy Choc Ice Cream

Serves: 2 kiddy serves
Preparation time: 5 minutes

Ingredients:
2 bananas, frozen, chopped
¼ cup milk, perferably Gabriel Method nut
milk (see page 256)
4 tsp cocoa powder
1 Tbsp flax seeds, ground
2 tsp protein powder
2 tsp xylitol if you require more sweetness
contents of 1 probiotic and 1 digestive
enzyme capsule (optional)

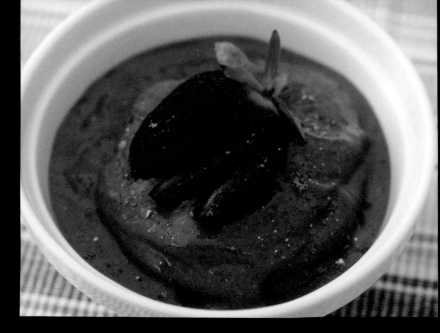

Method:
Place all ingredients in mixing jug. Blend together
with stick blender, ensuring all banana pieces are
thoroughly mixed through. Serve immediately

Gabrielicious Fudgesicle

Use the Easy Choc Ice Cream recipe to make Ice Cream
Pops or Fudgesicle. Using fresh bananas rather than frozen,
combine ingredients and distribute evenly into icy pole (popsicle)
moulds. Place in freezer for at least 3 hours or until set!

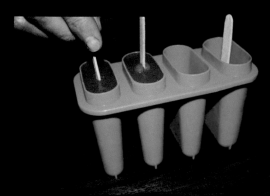

*"The Great American Fudgesicle -
Growing up as a kid my favourite
popsicle was called a fudgical. As
many of you know, it is a delicous,
smooth, creamy, chocolate treat.
It always put a smile on my face."*

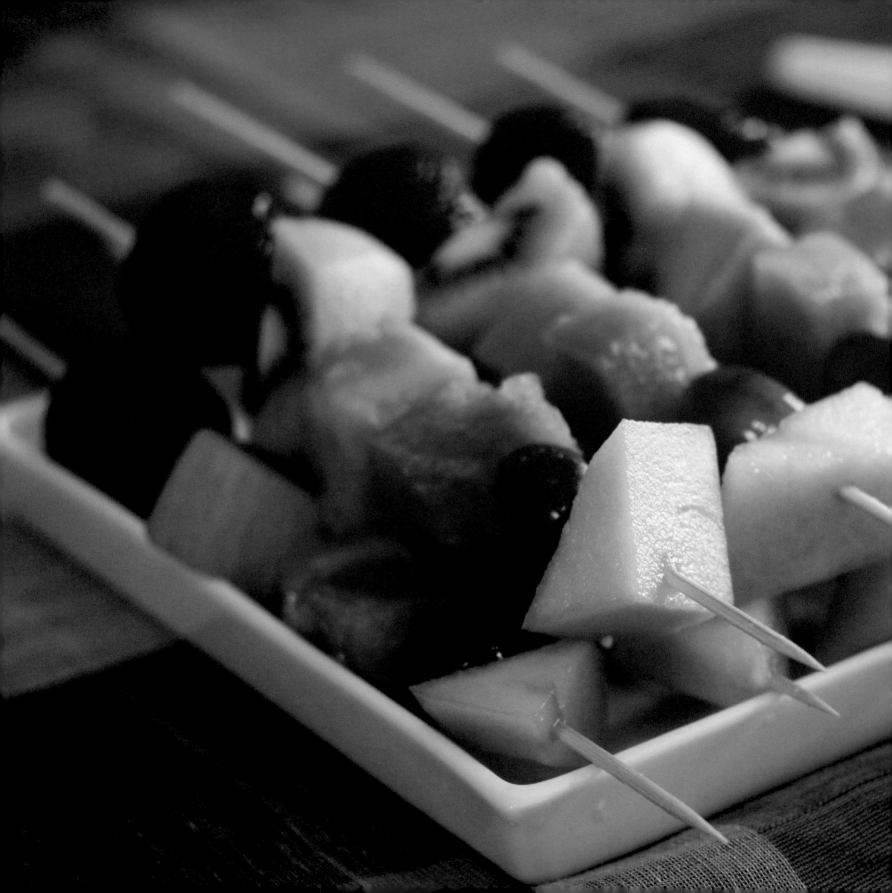

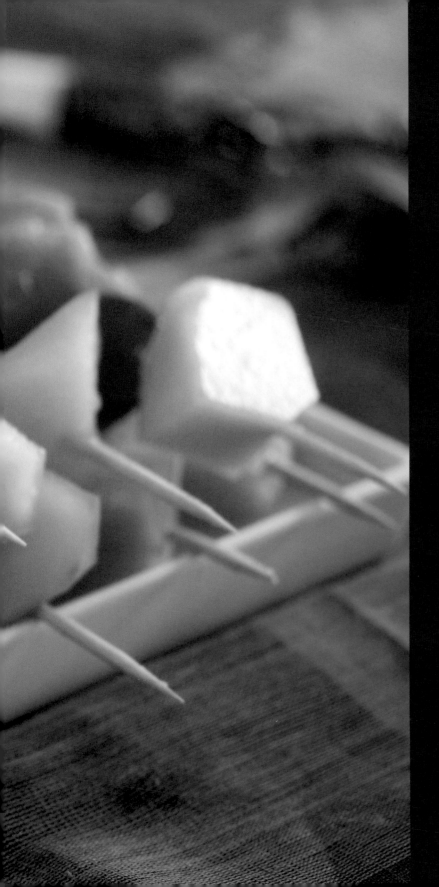

Fruit Kebabs

Makes: 10
Preparation time: 15 minutes

Ingredients:
10 strawberries
2 kiwi fruits
1 mango
¼ of a watermelon
¼ of a honeydew melon
10 red grapes

Method:
1. Cut all fruit into bite size chunks.
2. Thread the fruit pieces onto kebab sticks.
3. Refrigerate until ready to serve.

"I got this idea from a kiddy birthday party that my girlfriend hosted. She had all the standard sugary party foods but these fruit kebabs were the real hit. The kids loved them! There was something about fruit on a stick that was a real novelty for them and left them wanting more." - Oona

Almond and Orange Cake

Serves: 8
Preparation time: 20 minutes
Cooking time: 1 hour and 15 minutes

Ingredients:
2 oranges
1½ cups (240g) almonds
¾ cup xylitol
6 eggs (organic, free range)
1 teaspoon vanilla essence

Method:
1. Grease 20cm square cake tin, lining base with baking paper.
2. Place entire oranges (skins and all) in saucepan. Cover them with water and bring and cook. Once boiling, reduce heat and simmer for approximately 30 minutes or until skin has softened. Remove from water and allow to cool.
3. Preheat oven to 150°C / 300°F.
4. Blend almonds in food processor until coarsely chopped. Remove from food processor and set aside.
5. In food processor, place quartered unpeeled oranges. Blend until smooth. With motor running at low speed add eggs one at a time. Add almonds, xylitol and vanilla essence and continue to mix until combined.
6. Pour mixture into prepared pan and bake in oven for approximately 1 hour and 15 minutes or until cooked through.

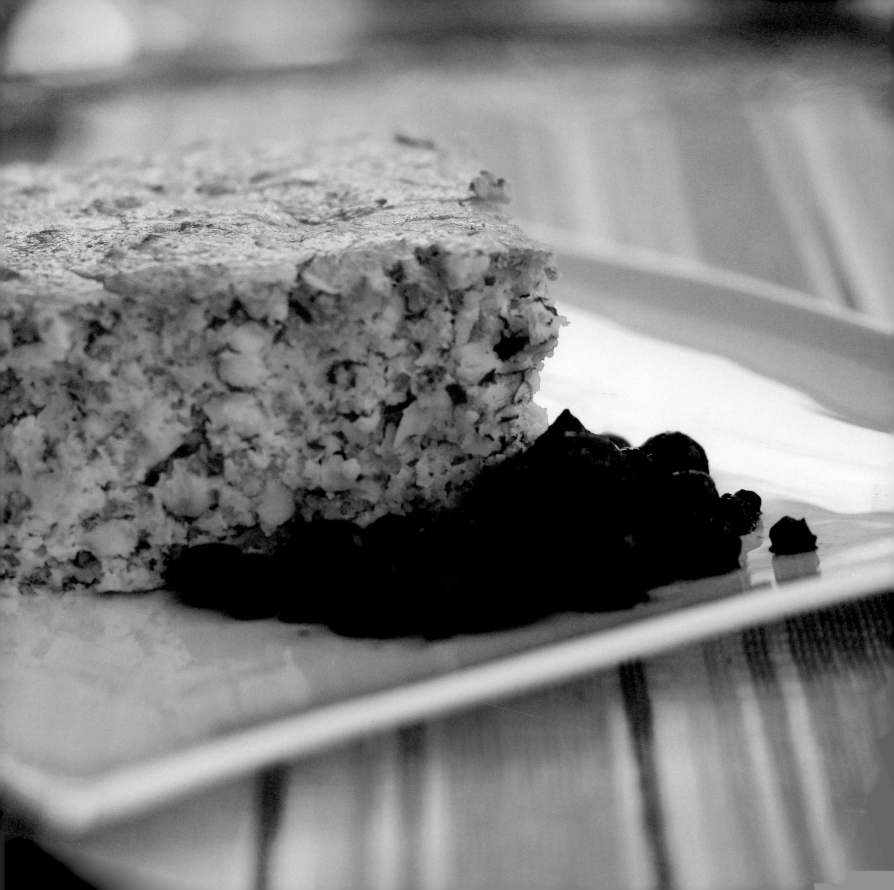

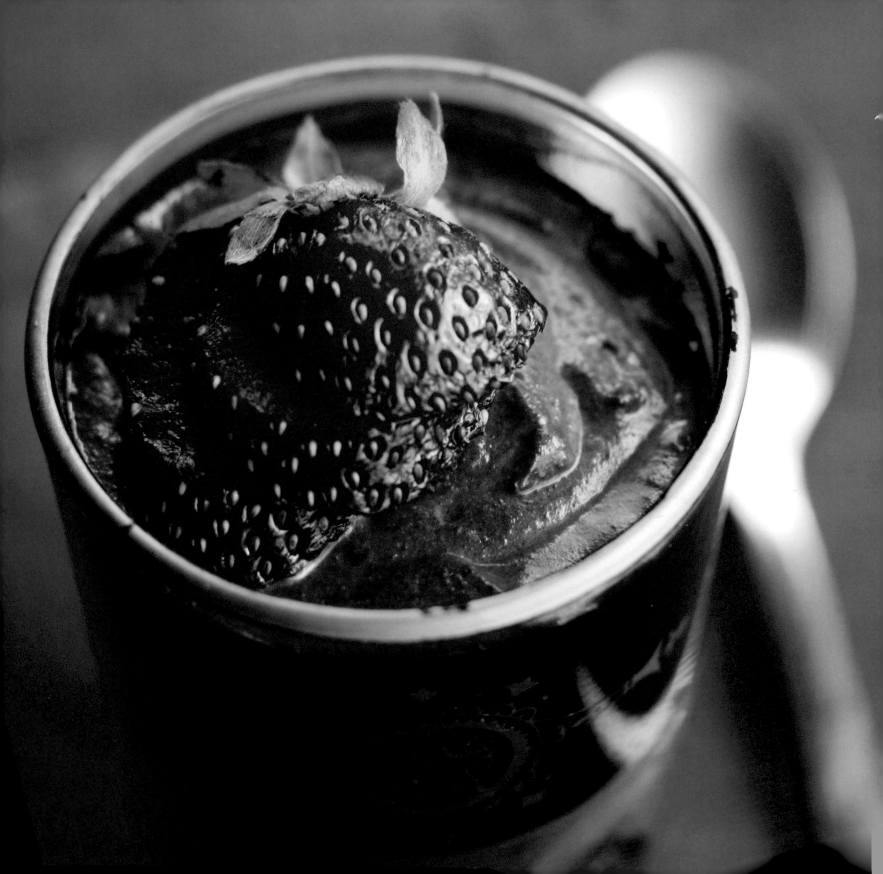

Chocolate Mousse

Serves: 6
Preparation time: 10 minutes
Setting time: 2 hours minimum

Ingredients:
250g ricotta cheese
4 Tbsp raw organic cocoa powder
3 Tbsp xylitol
3 Tbsp protein powder
4 egg yolks

Method:
1. Place ricotta into medium mixing bowl. Add cocoa powder, xylitol, protein powder and egg yolks. Stir to combine. To achieve an extra smooth consistency blend briefly with a stick blender.
2. Divide mixture among individual glasses or serving containers.
3. Place in fridge and allow to set for at least 2 hours.
4. Serve with fresh fruit, such as strawberries, and sprinkled with flax seeds.

"Creating this recipe was a moment of pure excitement for us, one of those brilliant inventions that comes out of a series of mistakes. While working on a healthy brownie recipe, we refrigerated some of the unused mixture and the result was incredible – perfect chocolate mousse.
We served this for the Gala Dinner Dessert at our Kiama Retreats and it brought the house down!"

Orange and Almond Cupcakes
with Chocolate Mousse Icing

Makes: 12
Preparation time: 20 minutes
Cooking time: 45 minutes

Ingredients:

2 small oranges (360g)
1½ cups (240g) almonds
½ cup xylitol

6 eggs (organic, free range)
1 teaspoon vanilla essence

Method:
1. Preheat oven to 150°C / 300°F. Place 12 cupcake holders into muffin tray.
2. Place entire oranges in saucepan. Cover them with water and cook. Once boiling, reduce heat to simmer for approximately 30 minutes or until skin has softened. Remove from water and allow to cool.
3. Blend almonds in food processor until coarsely chopped. Remove from food processor and set aside.
4. In food processor, place quartered oranges. Blend until smooth. With motor running at low speed add eggs one at a time. Add almonds, xylitol and vanilla essence and continue to mix until combined.
5. Pour mixture into prepared cup cake holders and bake in oven for approximately 45 minutes or until cooked through.

Chocolate Mousse Icing

Preparation time: 10 minutes

Ingredients:

125g ricotta
2 Tbsp raw organic cocoa powder
1½ Tbsp xylitol

1½ Tbsp protein powder
2 egg yolks

Method:
1. Place ricotta into medium mixing bowl. Add cocoa powder, xylitol, protein powder and egg yolks. Stir until well combined.
2. Ice each cupcake with a dollop of mixture.
3. Serve immediately or refrigerate to allow the mousse icing to set.

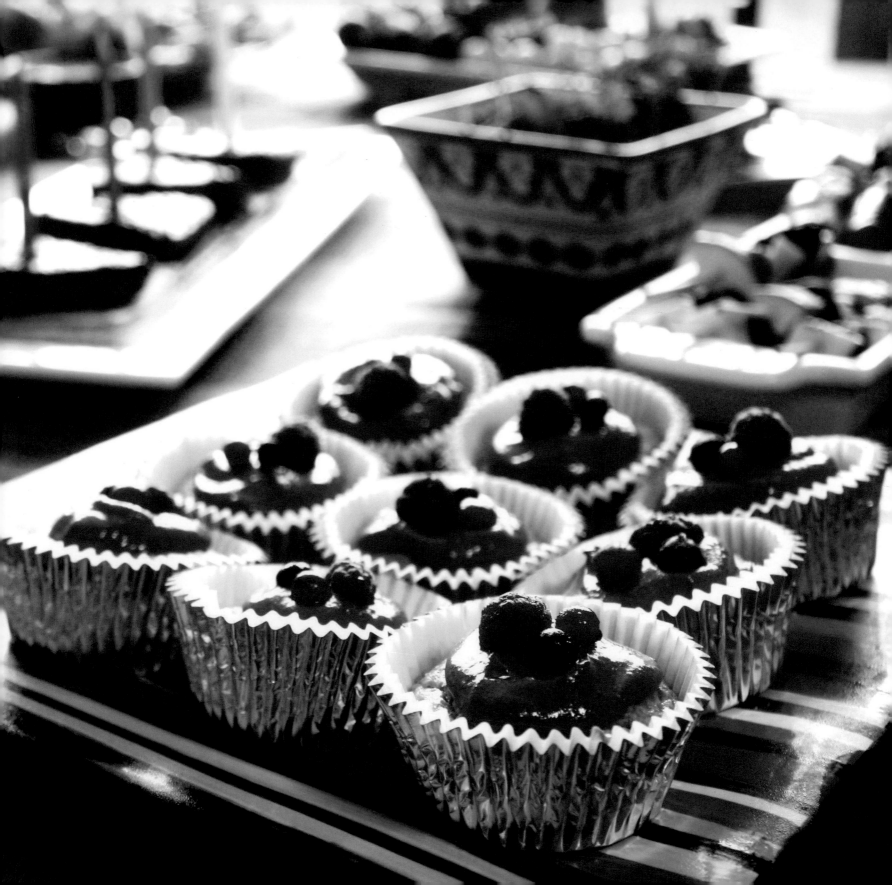

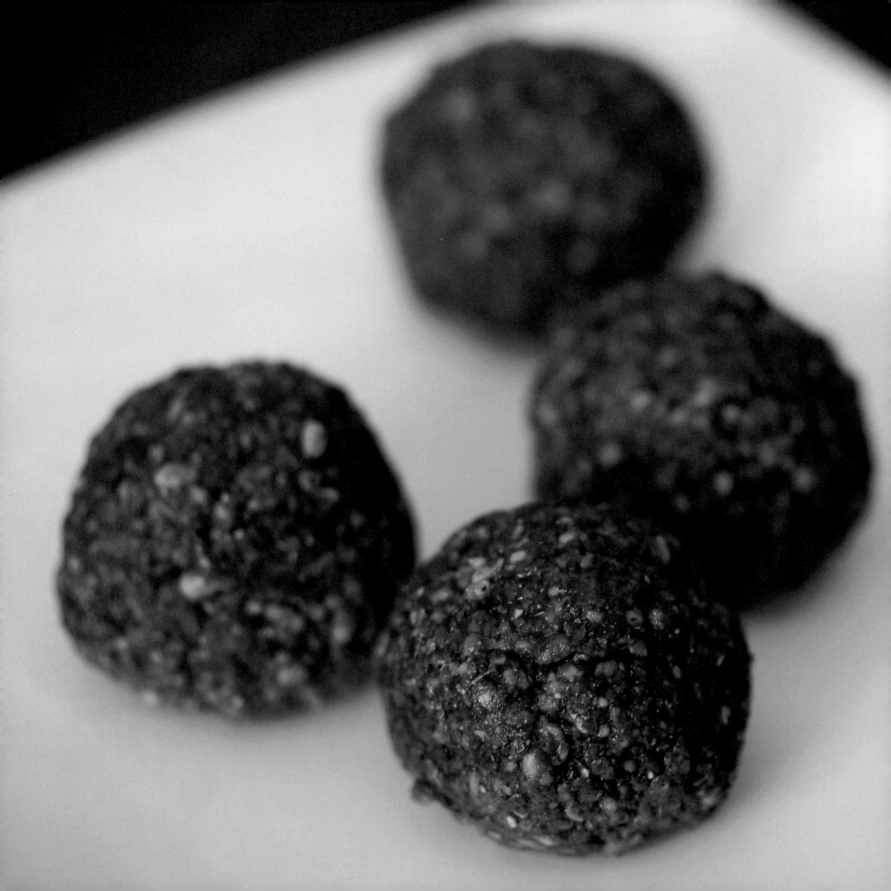

Raw Gingerbread Bites

Makes: 10
Preparation time: 15 minutes

Ingredients:
¼ cup flax seeds, ground
¼ cup walnuts
¼ cup almonds
2 tsp ground cinnamon
1 tsp ground ginger
¾ tsp ground cloves
2 tsp coconut palm sugar
1 tsp xylitol
2 Tbsp almond butter
1 Tbsp water

Method:
1. Place all dry ingredients into a food processor and process until well combined and beginning to stick together.
2. Add almond butter and water then blend until the mixture begins to stick together.
3. Form balls in the palms of your hands using approximately 1 tablespoon per ball.
4. Can be eaten immediately or refrigerated to allow to harden slightly.

Mini Ricotta Cheesecakes

Serves: 4
Preparation time: 15 minutes
Cooking time: 30 minutes

Ingredients:

For the base:
20g butter
¼ cup almonds
¼ cup sunflower seeds
¼ cup pepitas (pumpkin seeds)
¼ cup sesame seeds
¼ cup desiccated coconut
1 tsp coconut palm sugar

Crushed almonds to serve
Frozen berries to serve

For the filling:
2 eggs (organic, free range), separated
3 Tbsp xylitol
250g ricotta
rind of one lemon
2 Tbsp lemon juice
¼ cup plain yoghurt
1 tsp cinnamon
a pinch of stevia

Method:
1. Preheat oven to 180°C / 355°F.
2. Place all ingredients for the base in a food processor and process until coarsely ground.
3. Divide base mixture among 6 ramekins. Press down firmly with the back of a spoon.
4. In a medium bowl, beat egg whites until peaks form.
5. In a separate bowl, combine ricotta, lemon rind and juice, yoghurt, egg yolks, cinnamon, stevia and xylitol. Mix with electric mixer until you have achieved a smooth consistency.
6. Fold egg white mixture into ricotta mixture.
7. Distribute between ramekins and bake for 40 minutes.
8. Serve hot with crushed almonds and frozen berries.

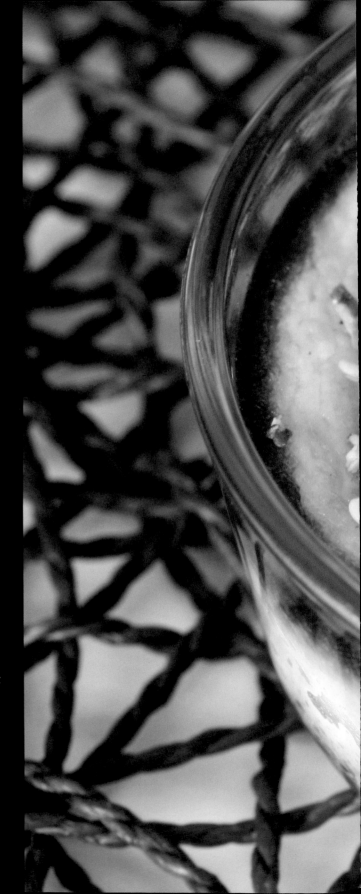

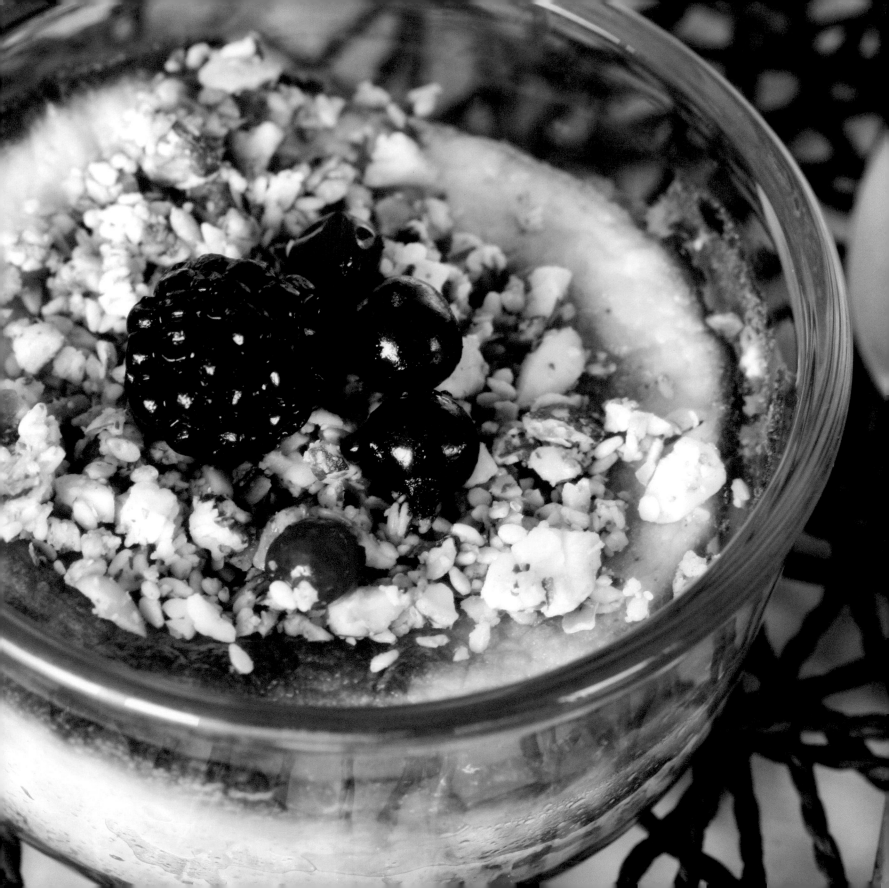

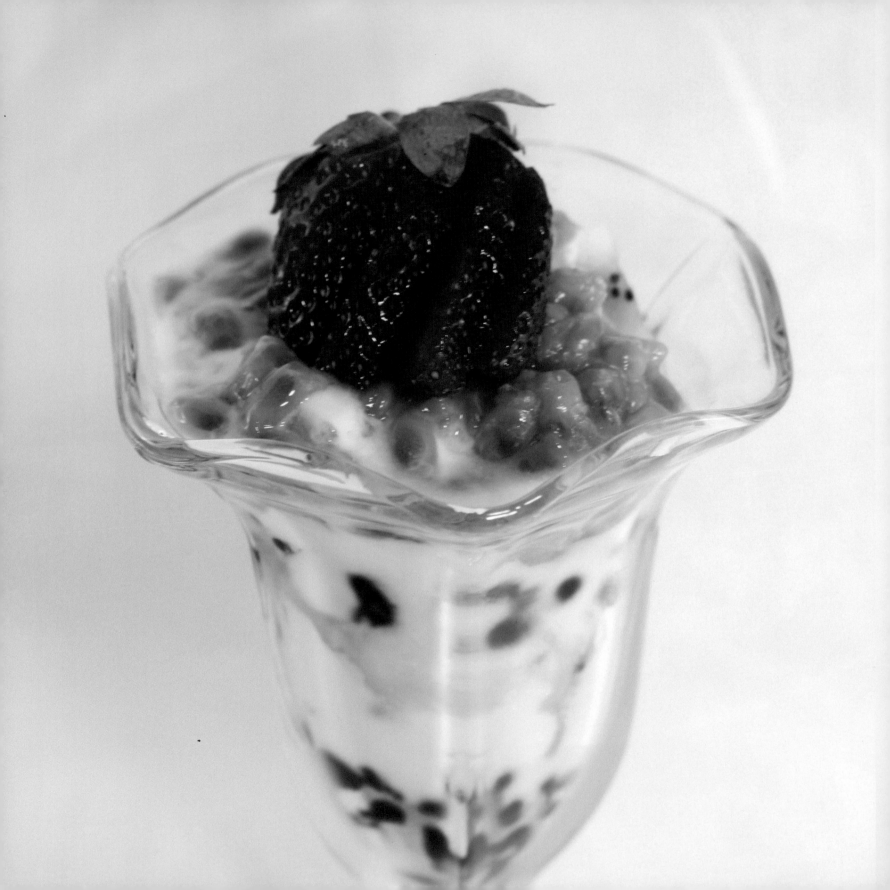

"This can be made with your choice of favourite fruits or seasonally available produce."

Fruit Parfait

Serves: 1
Preparation time: 5 minutes

Ingredients:
2 strawberries, halved
1 kiwi fruit,
½ passionfruit (approximately 2 Tbsp pulp)
4 Tbsp plain organic yoghurt
1 Tbsp flax seeds / chia seeds, ground
½ tsp xylitol, optional, to mix in to yoghurt before filling glass

Method:
Place strawberries at the bottom of the parfait glass and layer with 1 Tbsp yoghurt and a sprinkling of flax or chia seeds. Repeat this layering with other fruits until the glass is full. Top with passionfruit pulp. Sit back and enjoy the simple goodness.

I have been making and refining this recipe for months and months. There is an art to these brownies. The key is in the cooking process. Because there is no flour, the way these brownies cook and set is different to a conventional flour-based brownie but the effort is well worth your while.

Jonny's Chocolate Chia Crunch Brownies

Serves: 8
Preparation time: 10 minutes
Cooking time: 30 minutes
Cooling / Setting Time: 2 hour 15 minutes

Ingredients:
250g ricotta cheese
5 Tbsp unsweetened cocoa powder
6 eggs yolks
2 ½ Tbsp xylitol
2 ½ Tbsp coconut palm sugar
½ Tbsp chia seeds
¼ cup walnuts or hazelnuts, crushed

Method:
1. Pre-heat oven to 180°C / 355°F. Grease and line a bread loaf tin with baking paper.
2. Place all ingredients into a medium mixing bowl. Stir until well combined.
3. Pour mixture into loaf tin and bake in oven for 20 - 30 minutes. Check after 20 minutes. Insert a knife into the centre of the brownies. Take them out of oven when the sides are cooked but the centre is still slightly runny.
4. Allow brownies to sit for 15 minutes and then refrigerate for 2 hours to achieve a nice moist delicious brownie.

"This is a chocolate variation of our Orange and Almond cake – equally delicious!"

Jaffa Almond Cake

Makes: 8
Preparation time: 20 minutes + 30 minutes boiling
Cooking time: 1 hour 15 minutes

Ingredients:
2 small oranges (360g)
1½ cups almonds
½ cup xylitol
¼ cup coconut palm sugar
6 large eggs (organic, free range)
½ cup cocoa powder
1 tsp vanilla essence

Method:
1. Grease 20cm square cake tin, lining base with baking paper.
2. Place entire oranges in saucepan. Cover them with water and cook. Once boiling, reduce heat to allow to simmer for approximately 30 minutes or until skin has softened. Remove from water and allow to cool.
3. Preheat oven to 150°C / 300°F.
4. Blend almonds in food processor until coarsely chopped. Remove from food processor and set aside.
5. In food processor, place quartered oranges. Blend until smooth. With motor running at low speed add eggs one at a time. Add almonds, xylitol, coconut palm sugar, cocoa powder and vanilla essence and continue to mix until combined.
6. Pour mixture into prepared pan and bake in oven for approximately 1 hour and 15 minutes or until cooked through.

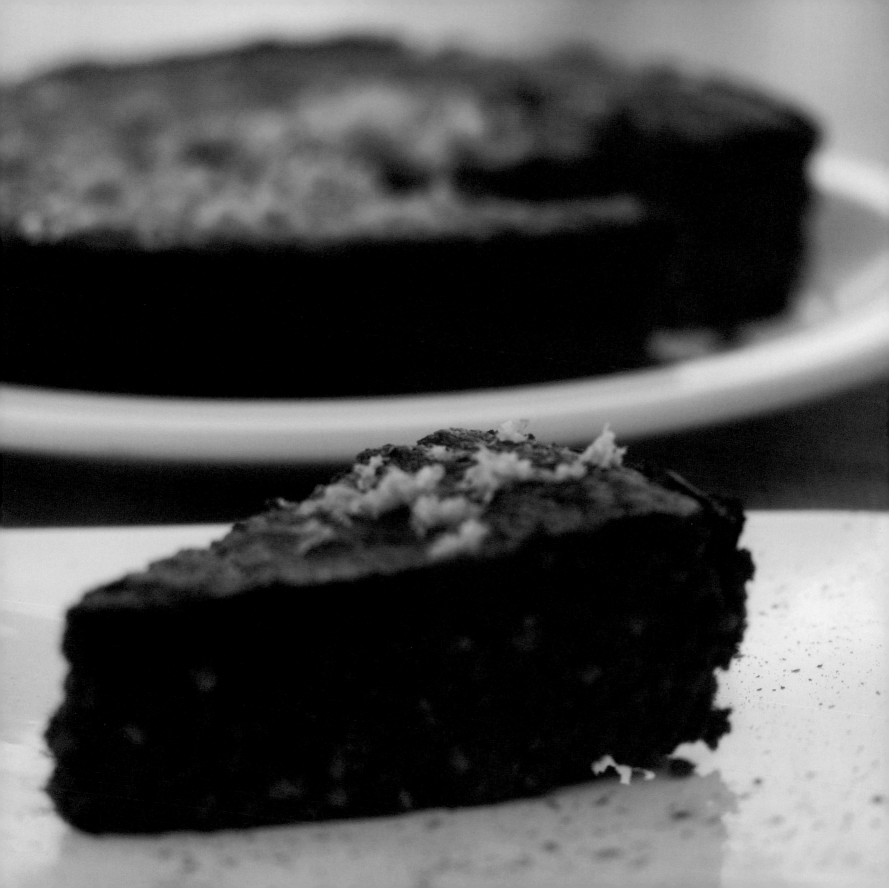

Watermelon Crush

Serves: 4
Preparation time: 10 minutes plus
3 hours freezing

Ingredients:
750g watermelon flesh, chopped
2 Tbsp lemon juice

Method:
1. Purée watermelon flesh in a food
   processor. Add lemon juice and
   stir through.
2. Place watermelon mixture into a
   freezer-safe container with a lid.
   Freeze for at least 3 hours.
3. Remove from freezer 10 minutes pri-
   or to serving. Remove lid and allow
   to thaw slightly. Mash with a fork.
   Place in glasses and serve. Even more
   refreshing when served with
   fresh mint.

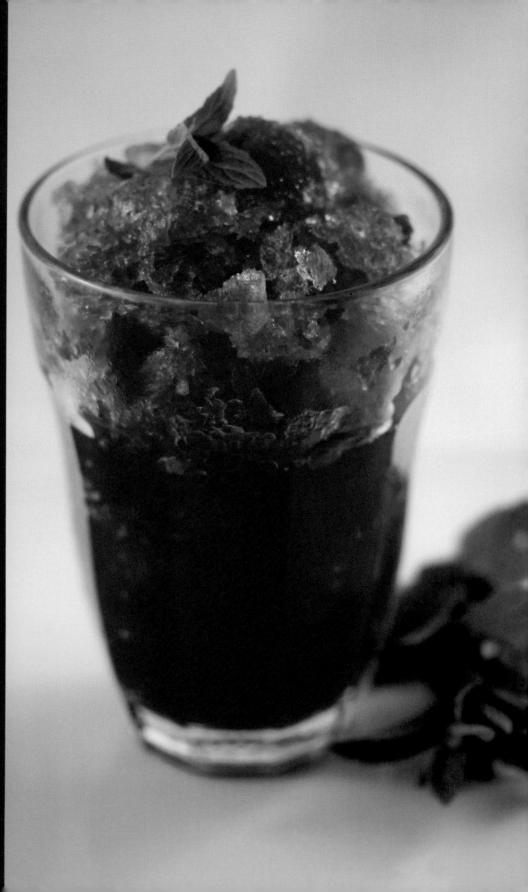

Lime Soda

Serves: 4
Preparation time: 5 minutes

Ingredients:
750mls sparkling mineral water
50ml lime juice
a pinch of stevia

Method:
Combine mineral water, lime juice and stevia. Stir together

"A great alternative to alcohol and sugar loaded soft drinks. Simply take it along to BBQs and picnics. Serve in a wine glass for more formal occasions."

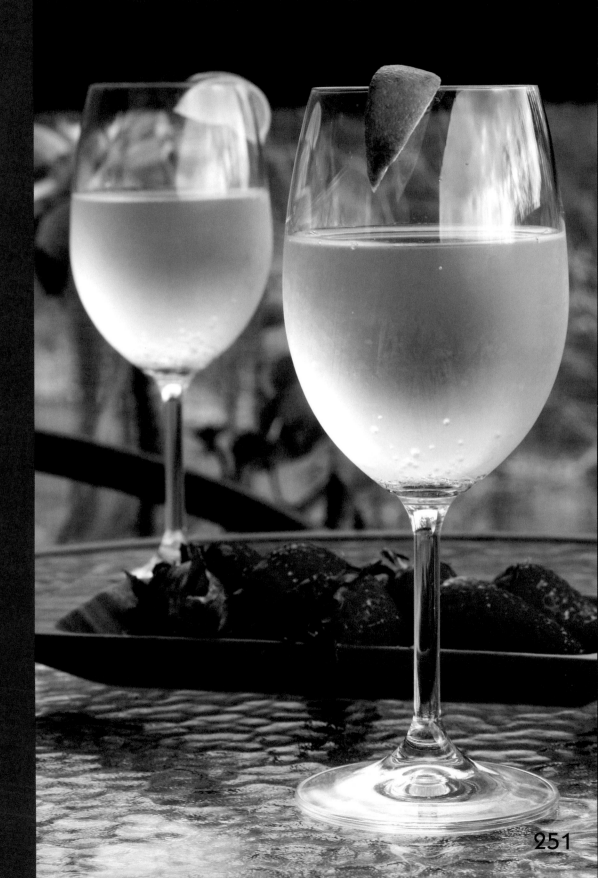

Frozen Fruit Slushie

Serves: 4
Preparation time: 5 minutes
Freezing time: 3 hours minimum

Ingredients:

¼ pineapple (approximately 330g), peeled, cored, chopped
1 orange, peeled, cored, chopped
¼ cup passionfruit pulp
2 Tbsp flax seeds, ground
2 Tbsp protein powder

Method:

1. Place all ingredients in food processor and process until smooth.
2. Pour entire contents into an airtight container and place in the freezer.
3. Freeze for a minimum of 3 hours. Remove from freezer and mash contents with a fork. If you have left it in freezer longer than 3 hours you will need to allow time for thawing before serving. You want a slushie icy consistency.
4. Distribute evenly between 4 glasses and serve.

A great refreshing summer drink that the whole family will love – with all of The Gabriel Method Big 3s.

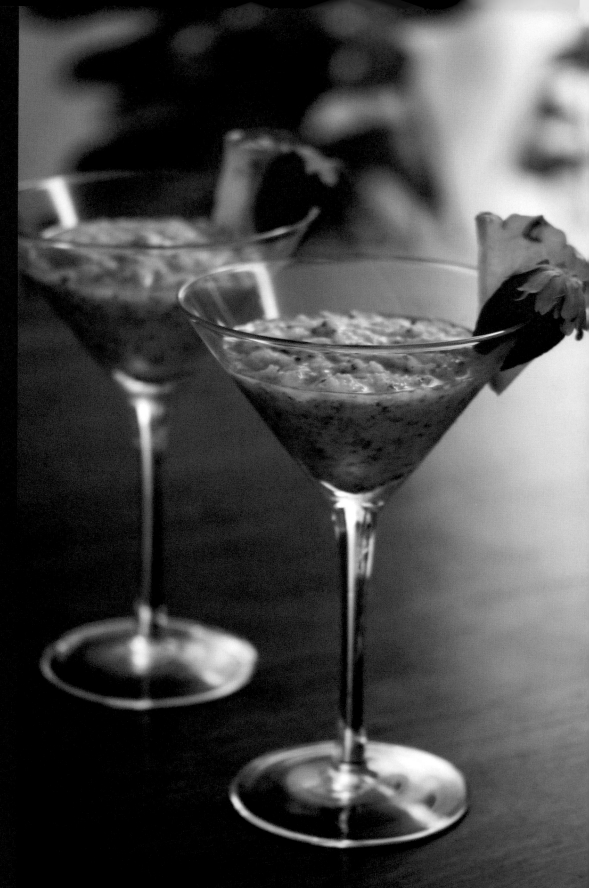

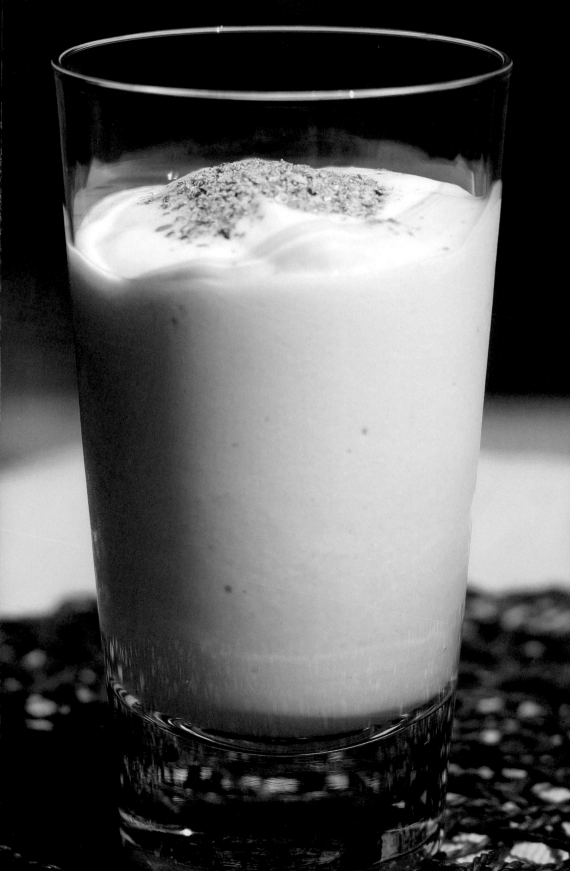

"This is a Gabriel Method version of the traditional Indian drink, and every bit as delicious. Perfect with a hot curry or simply as a refreshing drink."

Mango Lassi

Serves: 1
Preparation time: 5 minutes

Ingredients:
1 frozen mango cheek, cubed
¾ cup yoghurt
ground flax seeds to serve

Method:
Place mango and yoghurt together in mixing jug. Blend with stick blender until all of the mango is blended through. Pour into glass, sprinkle with flax seeds and serve.

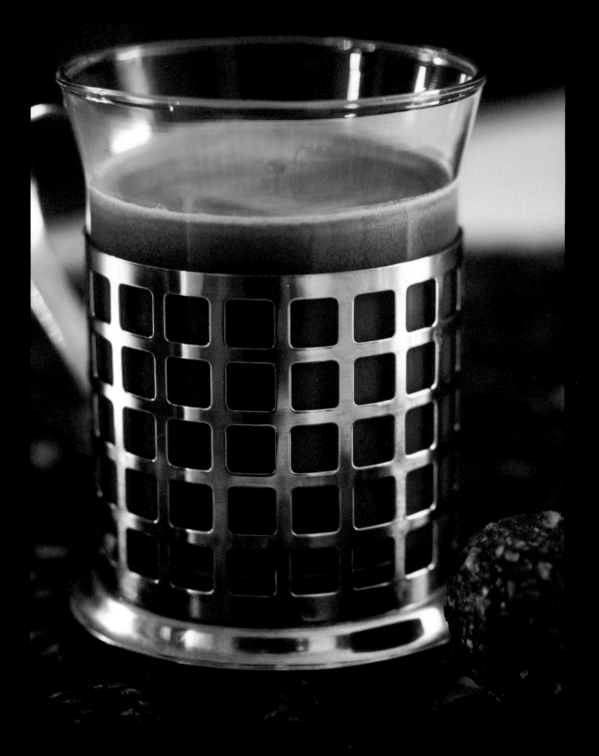

"Your kids will love this hot chocolate, as will their bodies."

Gabriel Method Hot Chocolate

Serves: 1
Preparation time: 5 minutes

Ingredients:
3 tsp cocoa powder
1 tsp protein powder
2 tsp coconut palm sugar
¼ cup almond milk (or milk of your choice)
¾ cup boiled water

Method:
1. Place all ingredients, except water, in mixing jug. Blend together with stick blender until you achieve a smooth consistency.
2. Pour into your favourite mug. Add hot water. Serve instantly.

Variations:
Maca Hot Choc:
Follow the basic recipe, adding ½ tsp maca powder to mixing jug prior to blending.

Cinnamon Hot Choc:
Follow the basic recipe, adding 1 tsp cinnamon to mixing jug prior to blending.

Chilli Hot Choc:
Follow the basic recipe, adding pinch of chilli powder to mixing jug prior to blending.

Gabriel Method Nut Milk

Makes: 1 litre
Preparation time: 5 minutes
Soak time: 4 hours minimum

Ingredients:
¾ cup raw organic almonds
½ cup raw organic Sunflower seeds (optional)
5 cups water
a pinch of stevia
1 Tbsp coconut palm sugar
a pinch of healthy salt
cheese cloth, unbleached

Method:
1. Soak almond and sunflower seeds in water for a minimum 4 hours, or overnight.
2. Place nut mixture into mixing jug. Thoroughly grind using a stick blender.
3. Place cheese cloth over jug. Tip upside down over a bowl to allow liquid to strain through cloth. Squeeze cheese cloth to get the remaining liquid out.*
4. Add stevia, salt and coconut palm sugar. Stir to combine.
5. Drink immediately or refrigerate.

*Save the nut pulp and use it with our Almond Chicken recipe (see page 145).

A tasty, healthy milk. Great for drinking on its own or for use in Gabriel Method smoothies, ice creams, mueslis, desserts or as a substitue for dairy milk in any other recipe.

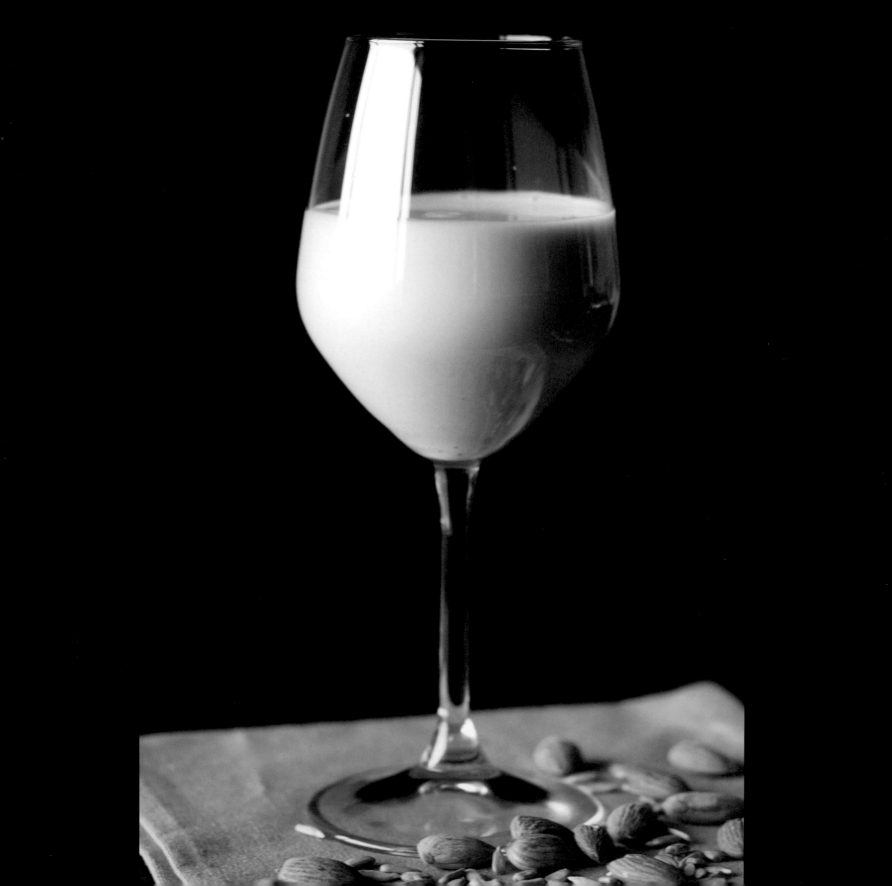

Pinada Colada

Makes: 1 litre
Preparation time: 10 minutes

Ingredients:
1 very ripe pineapple, peeled,
cored and cubed*
1 cup coconut milk
6 Tbsp lime juice
Ice cubes to serve

*The ripeness of your pineapple
makes all the difference between
a bitter and sweet piña colada!

Method:
1. Place all ingredients in food
    processor and process until
    well combined.
2. Serve with ice cubes

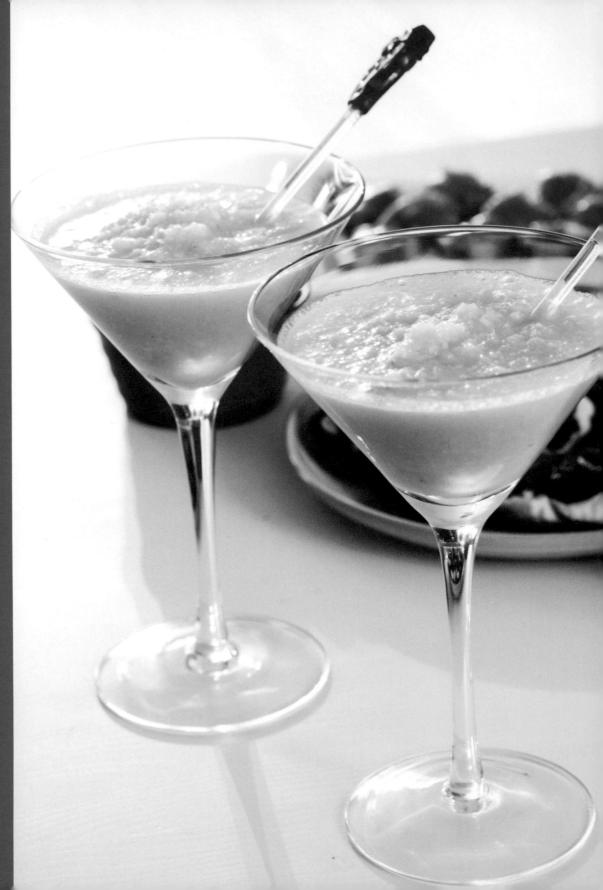

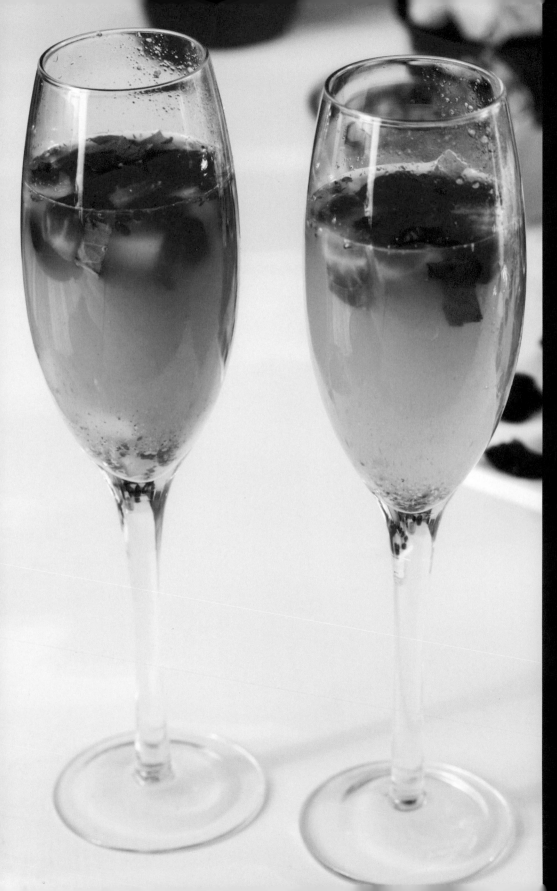

Fruit Punch

Makes: 3 litres
Preparation time: 5 minutes

Ingredients:
2 litres sparkling mineral water
1 litre freshly squeezed orange juice
½ cup lime juice
225g pineapple, cut into small chunks
100g strawberries, chopped into
small pieces
1 Tbsp flax seeds, ground
10 fresh mint leaves

Method:
1. Place all liquid ingredients into a large bowl that you will serve your punch in.
2. Add fruit, flax seeds and mint.
3. Add ice cubes prior to serving. Use a spouted ladle to pour into glasses.

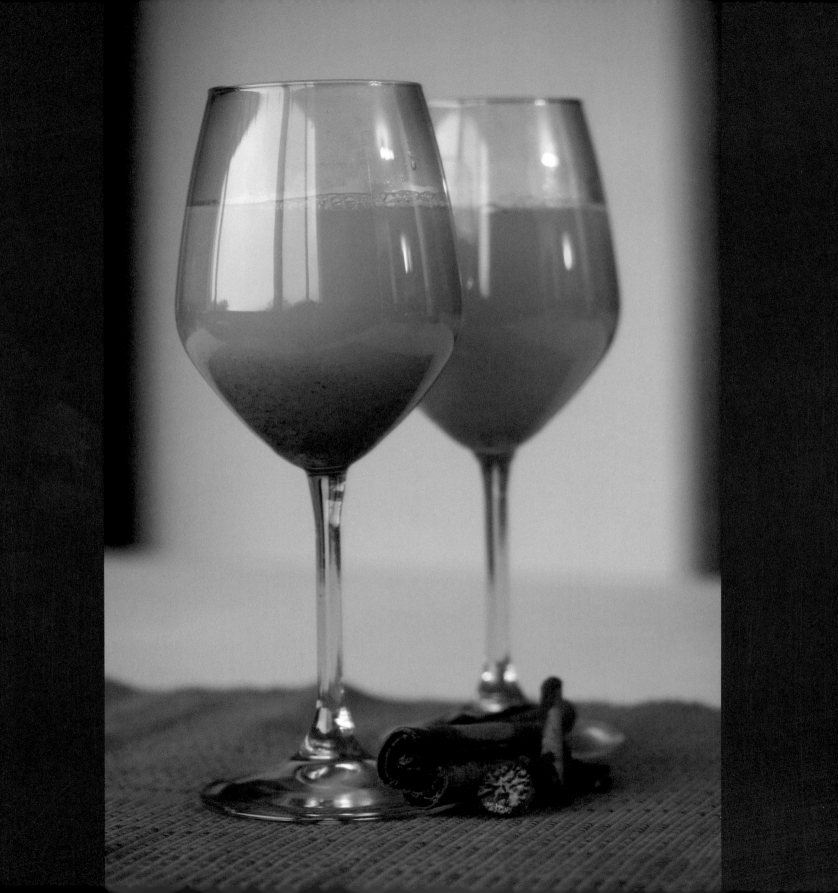

Warm 'n Spicy Apple Cider

Serves: 1.5 litres
Preparation time: 10 minutes
Cooking time: 10 minutes

Ingredients:
4 cups water
4 oranges, freshly juiced (approximately ⅔ cup)
juice of 2 lemons (approximately ¼ cup)
20 whole cloves
6 cinnamon quills
1 nutmeg, grated
4 apples
4 slices ginger

Method:
1. In a large saucepan on high heat, combine water, orange juice, lemon juice, cloves, cinnamon and nutmeg. Allow to boil for 5 minutes. Reduce heat to low and simmer.
2. In your juicer, juice the apples and ginger. Set aside.
3. Remove spice mix from heat and strain into a serving jug or pot.
4. Add apple and ginger juice. Serve warm.

Entertaining

Eating is one of the most universal ways of being social. You can find the principle of 'eat, drink and be merry' across all cultures and times.

This is especially true for holidays and celebrations. The good news is that you can Gabrielise even the most decadent and indulgent of feasts simply by applying The Gabriel Method principles to your treats to make them even more delicious and nutritious. For adults, cocktails can become "mocktails" and for the kids cakes and ice cream can still be "Gabrielicious".

To make entertaining the Gabriel way easy for you, in this section we've gathered together plenty of ideas to get you started. With quick and easy reference guides to the recipes that we feel will do your party justice.

Having healthy fun doesn't mean having to compromise on flavour or presentation.

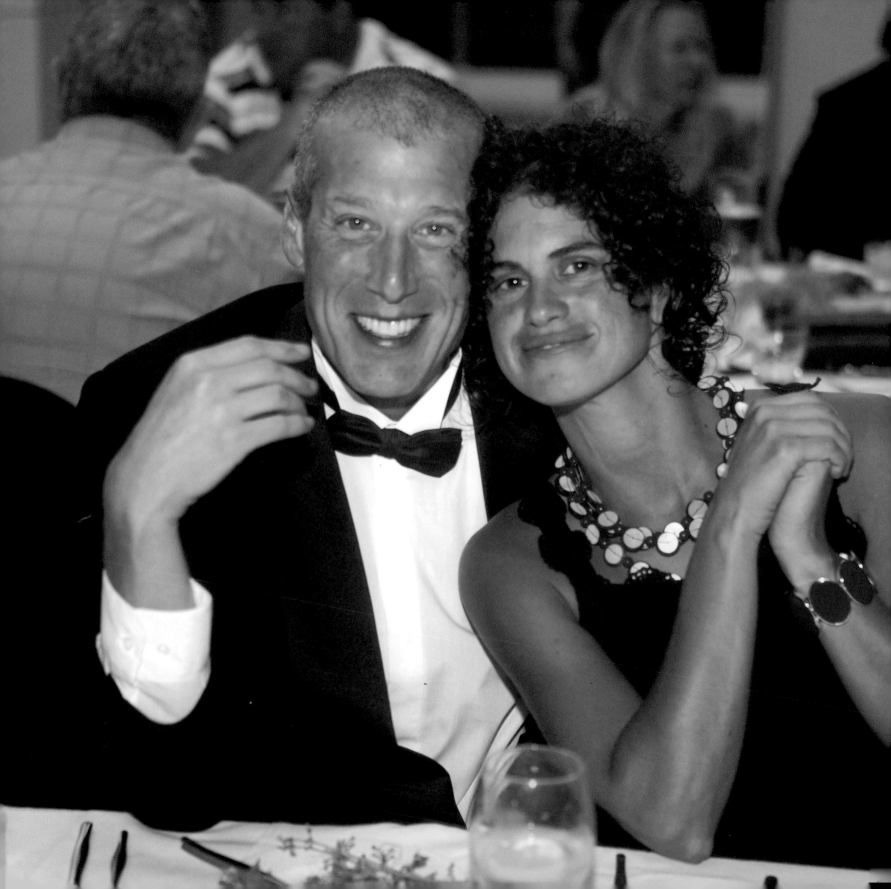

Kids' Parties

"Imagine a kid's party without the sugar-high manias followed by the 'inevitable' sugar-crash tantrums! Well, now you don't have to, because when you hold a kids' party the Gabriel way you know that the kids will love the food and they'll be a little more even-keeled, thus keeping your sanity intact. Well, mostly ..."

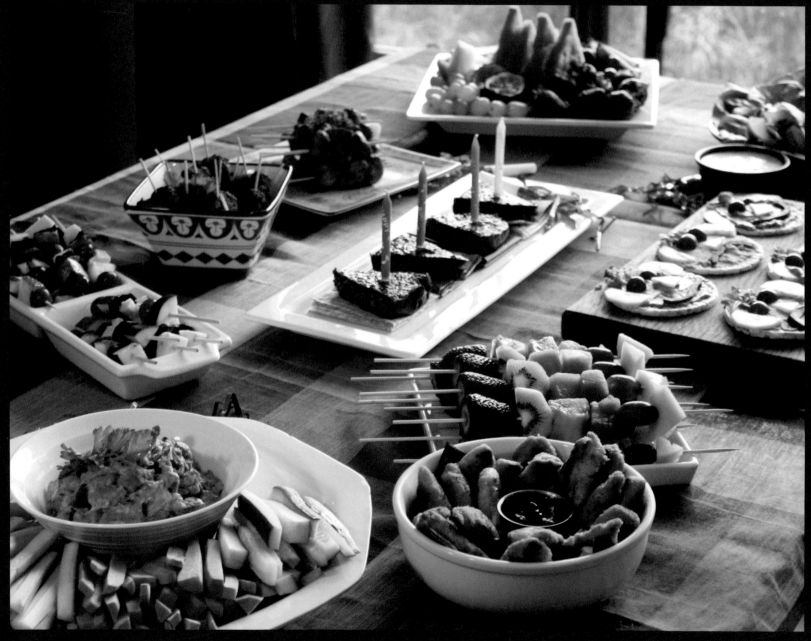

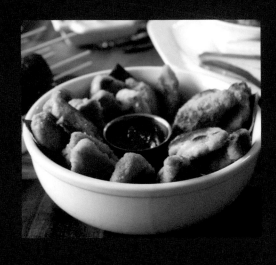

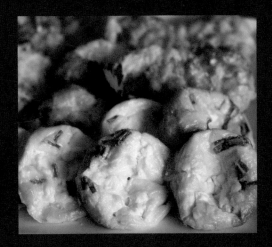

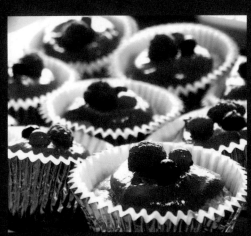

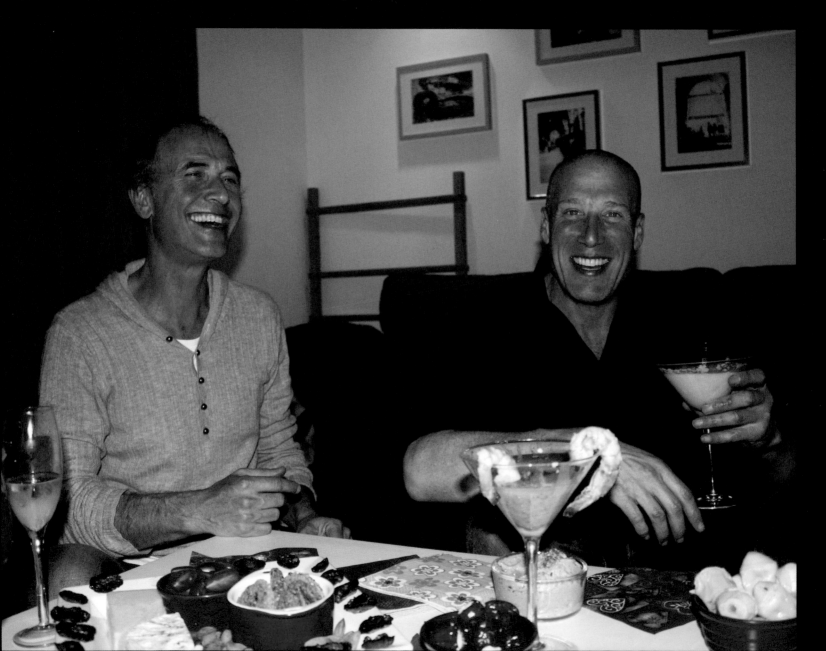

"A great opportunity to get together with friends! And what better way to play than letting out that inner alchemist and devising delightful concoctions."

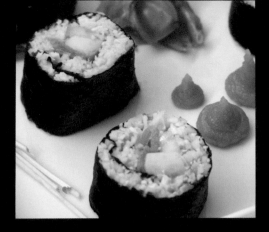

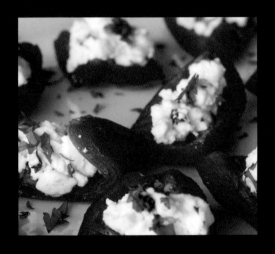

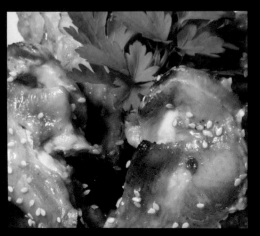

Barbecue

"The great summer institution of the barbecue was made for healthy eating. Everything's about salads and protein and in a spirit of adventure you can find whole new worlds of flavours, scents and colours to entertain yourselves and your guests."

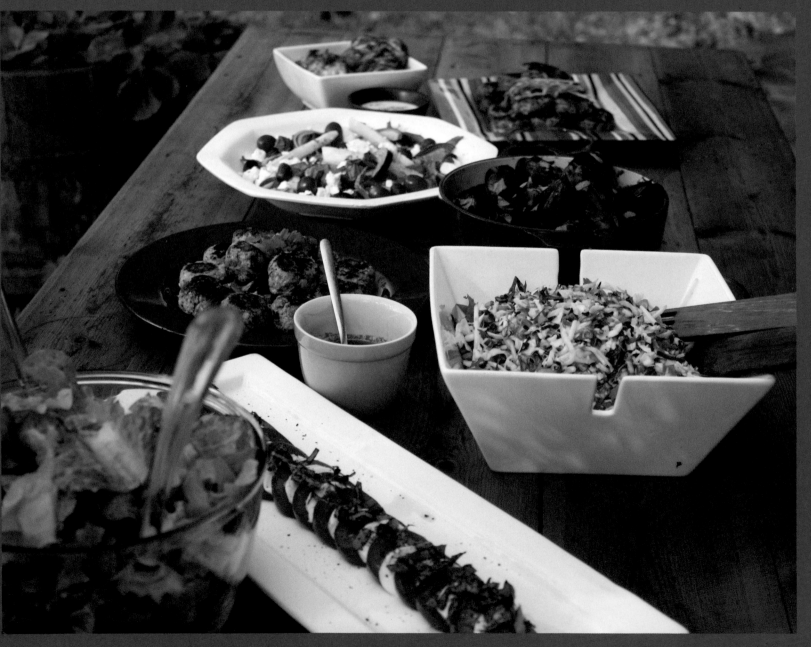

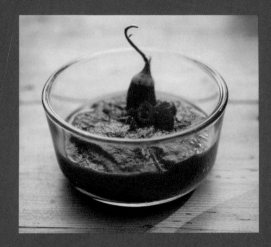

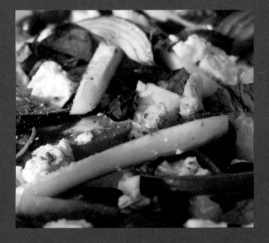

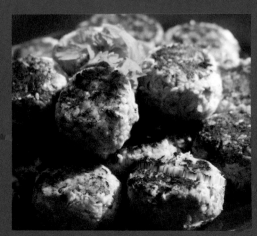

Christmas

"Ahhh, Christmas, the season of indulgence and the great enemy of the dieter. Fortunately, The Gabriel Method is not a diet, so as long as you stick to the principles, eat up! This is not the time to deprive yourself of anything. Your body will tell you when you've had enough anyway."

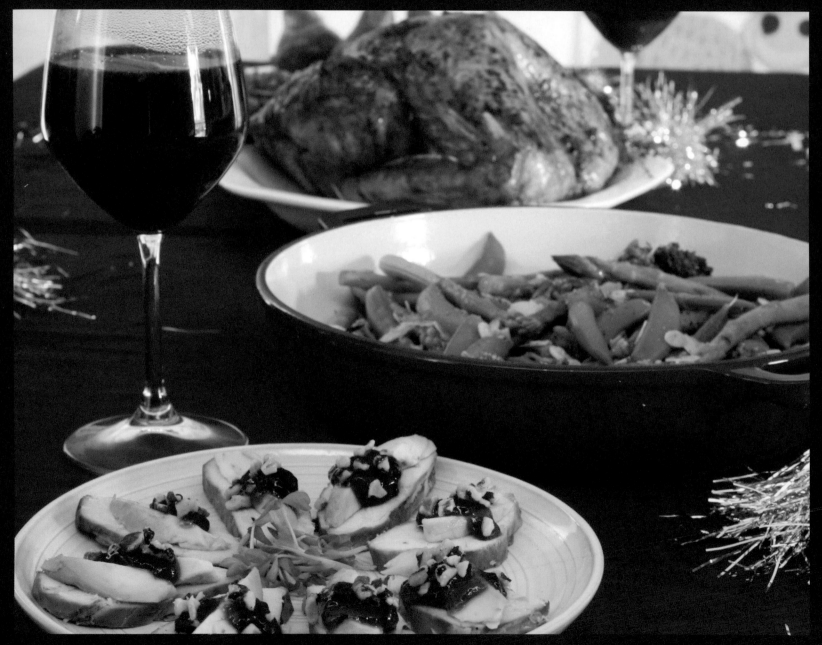

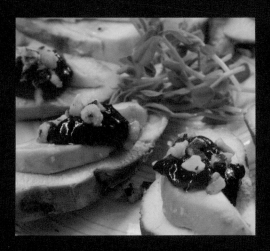

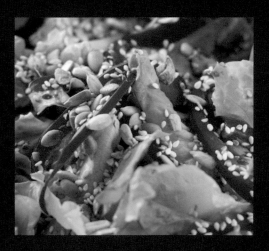

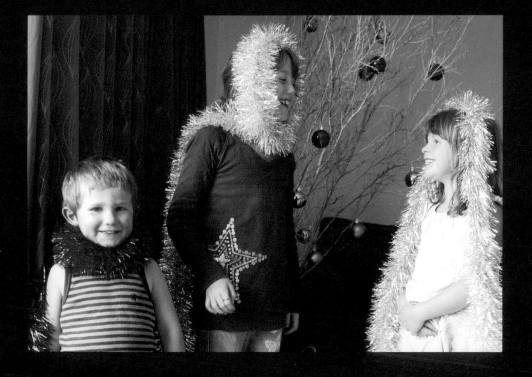

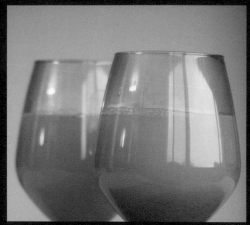

Acknowledgements

There are so many people that have helped in the formation and creation of this recipe book, that I don't think I could possibly name all of them. But just to name a few...

First and foremost I'm greatly indebted to Oona for her tireless effort, her passion and her creative brilliance with recipe design and food photography. Biggest ever thanks to Teegan O'Hehir for her inspiration with recipes, creativity and necessary bossiness in the kitchen. I'd also like to thank Kelly Jones for her beautiful designs and remarkable patience; Nic Duncan for the gorgeous cover shot and lifestyle pics; Xavier Waterkeyn for his editing genius (yes I know the word 'genius' does not do you justice, X, I'm sorry, they just haven't made a better word for what you do. Don't blame me, it's the English language's fault). Sharon Humphreys, Lydia Kenyon, and Judith Bradley for their equally brilliant editing assistance; Lucas Rockwood and his team for their tireless efforts; Bernadette, Wadie and Julia Mansour, Emma Shea, Tamala, Sabine, Nikki, Jenny and Ethel for recipe inspiration. Thanks to Gabbys catering, in Kiama, for bringing our recipes to life for so many people.

Thanks to our many tasters – Sabine, Jonno, Melinda, Augy, Isla, Mum, Julia, Simon, Zen, Sapphire, Tyce, Serena, Gadi and Lalita, Tam, Brian and Jethro - for their eagerness and honesty. Thanks to our local suppliers of top quality produce: Reeves Butchers, Denmark Health Shop and Denmark's IGA Express.

And my deepest appreciation to Jenny, Shannon, Aeron, Helen, Cherie and Cheryl from my office, Jack Strom and Marjolijn Loderichs; Rafi Nasser and Robert Peng for their inspiration; Phan, Prajnananda, Khaliah Ali, Joey, Jennifer and Ethel Abrams. And the thousands of people on my forums and seminars that have aided in the creating and perfecting of these recipes. I am so grateful to you all for being in my life and helping me bring this vision into a reality.

Eternal thanks to 3 incredibly special beings - Inge, Maya and Xabi - for being the biggest inspiration and most honest critiques any cook could ever ask for.

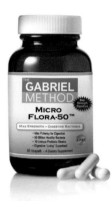
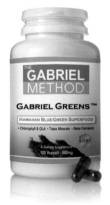
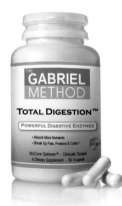
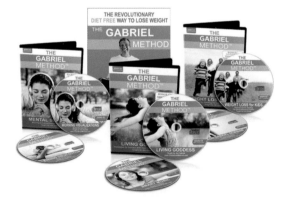